The Healing Point

A step by step formula to help you find more energy, overcome sickness, and become a healthier version of you.

James Lilley

Health has
no value till
sickness
comes

Thomas Fuller

Table of Contents

Disclaimer: Every effort has been made to ensure that the information contained in this book is complete and accurate. The statements made in this book have not been evaluated by the U.S. Food and Drug Administration (FDA). The products mentioned in this book are not intended to treat, diagnose, cure, or prevent any disease. The information provided in this book is not a substitute for a consultation with your own physician, and should not be construed as individual medical advice. Although this book contains information relating to health care, the information is not intended as medical advice and is not intended to replace a person-to-person relationship with a qualified healthcare professional. If you know or suspect you have a health problem, it is recommended that you first seek the advice of a physician before trying out any medical program or treatment. All efforts have been made to assure the accuracy of the information contained in this book at the time of publication. The author disclaims any liability for any medical outcomes that may occur as a result of applying the methods suggested in this book.

This is a must read! Recommending it to all my clients!!!
I have sat with this masterpiece, reading it from cover to cover in its entirety, twice now. I have not been able to put it down, between the warm delivery of this work, and the endless re-invigoration of information offered. This book does what others have yet to do, and that is to break down a most complicated issue of acute to chronic illness into an easily read, yet impeccably researched guide to the foundation of health and HOW to be the picture of health.

With drug companies lining the pockets of the medial world, and doctors in patient's purses, James has stripped away the fog blinding us, while revealing through well documents accounts of a personal, treacherous, endured course of what was once, and could have been, a slow an arduous death. James delivers a wealth of knowledge through a conversation that feels like an invitation to tea, while he reveals the meaning of health and how to achieve your optimal state.

What is more, is that there are no products, supplements, programs, or additional books being pushed or offered; but an empowering and comprehensive roadmap placing you in the driver's seat of your own body. From cellular foundations of health and disease to home testing of organ functions, nutrition, and rebalancing what has been off-kilter, these short chapters are easy to navigate with interactive invitations to help you become your own expert and take charge of your health. This will literally be the only book you will ever need for staying healthy and disease free the rest of your life.

Top customer reviews

SO Much More Than a Health Book

The first thing that you notice about The Healing Point is its striking cover. As you start reading you realize this is not a typical health book.

The introduction sets the tone for the whole book. The author's chatty voice makes everything easy to understand. This strong authors voice continues throughout the book. The author avoids too much jargon. His antidotes make everything easy to understand. There are scenarios the author poses to the reader which make you think.

The book contains information about several products and diets. There are no product links and nothing is oversold. With all the information the author never seems to preach. Instead, he gives the information and lets the reader make their own decisions.

I remember thinking halfway through the book. Blimey, I'm actually enjoying a health book. This is not a health book it is so much more. There are parts that include the author's own story. This makes the book so much better to read. When you see the motivation behind a book you pay it more attention.

This book is an absolute must-read for all, regardless if you are ill or not. The amount of information contained in this book will need revisiting several times. I suggest you buy your own copy as this is a book you will want to read again and again.

.

Top customer reviews

Your roadmap to health is here!!!

I am VERY impressed by the clarity, coherency, and compassion of this book. When you are ready to take personal responsibility for your own health you will find this book to be an invaluable asset. This book features dozens of well-researched, easy to implement health strategies for directing your own personal path to health and happiness. This is a heartfelt and inspiring work. Do yourself a favor and buy it! Your good health is in your hands!

Top customer reviews

A great resource for anyone looking for abundant life

Thank you James for writing this book. You have consolidated the material of many authors I have previously read, and your writing has distilled it down to a readable recipe for a lifestyle that offers hope, encouragement, and sustainability for a long and rewarding life.

Top customer reviews

A friend recommended this book to me

It is an easy read and Mr. Lilley is quite funny. He writes his story in such a way that I want to follow his suggestions. I also finished the book in two days. It was akin to reading a health book in a story. Anyway, it worked for me, I started the mini cleanse and four days into it, I am still doing it. I have recommended the book to several family members and, btw, this is my first review.

Top customer reviews

I loved EVERYTHING about this amazing book

I have owned and run my own health food store for over 24 years and this is a book I will recommend to ALL my customers. James is straight to the point and because of his personal health struggles has so much insight as to the REAL issues. Love, love, love this book

Top customer reviews

One of the most influential books I have read!!!

First let me say I have never read a "health" book before. This was not just a book about someone telling you that you HAVE to live your life a certain way. This book makes you look at everything in a very different perspective. The author brings us into his struggles (which we all have in one way or another) and talks through his book as if he is talking one on one with a friend. This was a fantastic read and I strongly suggest anyone reading it.

Top customer reviews

Detailed with bonus links and lots of info.

Well composed and well written. Clearly a lot of attention paid to not only the content but also the presentation. In depth personal experiences together with diet explanations and teachings on the inner workings of our bodies. Would recommend to anyone who wants to better understand how what we put into our bodies impacts more than just how full we feel.

13

Introduction

Hi, I'm James.

For the past two years this book has quietly burned inside me like an incessant obsession, this wasn't the story I intended to tell, and yet here we are, staring each other firmly in the eye.

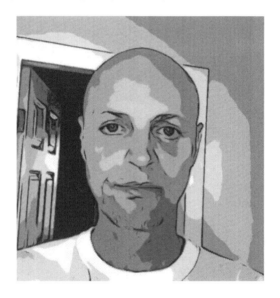

To keep things interesting, cutting edge information is presented in a relaxed style with warmth and compassion — almost like two old friends chatting over a pot of tea. Along the way, there may be times when we laugh together in the face of adversity, and perhaps even share a moment or two of profound sadness.

Either way, I aim to provide you with engaging content that's enjoyable to read. I think you will find my style refreshingly simple and authentic. Thanks for stopping by and I hope you enjoy what I have to offer.

Chapter 1

CAUGHT WITHOUT A PLAN

There could be many reasons why you picked up this book. Perhaps your goal is to have more energy, better mental clarity, or you simply come in search of tools to help you overcome a stubborn illness. Let's explore that last option first, and then work our way backward.

Illness is a puzzle; to try to solve it we first need to understand it. Typically, there are two ways to do this. The first is to enlist the services of a medical professional. This approach is not without merit, but it often involves taking medications. Perhaps you have already tried this route and have yet to find a lasting solution.

The second option is to stop what you are doing and listen. Do you hear them? Those annoying symptoms we sometimes complain about are an effective system of communication. They are your body's way of letting you know something you are doing sucks. Until now, you may not have been paying close attention. That's okay because your body is sure to send you a much clearer signal soon.

The medical term for that signal is pain.

Pain lets us know there is a problem in the body. The same way a vehicle check engine light might alert us to a problem under the hood. The key to improving health is learning to listen to your symptoms. This is how medicine was practiced for thousands of years long before illness became a lucrative industry.

Symptoms offer important clues which in turn help us to find lasting solutions. Unfortunately, many of these clues are often silenced by prescription drugs such as painkillers.

I suspect if the prescription drug approach had worked for you in the past, then you wouldn't be reading this book. For some, drugs do little to address the root cause of the problem. And so the underlying health problem rarely goes away.

At this point, it's worth noting that certain prescription drugs have been known to cause serious side effects and even death! Some estimates put the figure at over 100,000 deaths per year. That's twice as many Americans who die from prescription drugs than are killed in car accidents. To simplify: you take a pill to feel better, but then you die. *What's up with that?*

It's a worry that should be commanding front page news. But instead, we fill our news with the mundane gossip of celebrities we will never meet. We then face a slick, billion-dollar industry that offers us hope and side effects in the same TV commercial.

In the interest of fairness, I'd also like to point out that there *are* FDA approved drugs that deliver lifesaving benefits. And for some, a visit to the doctor may even bring immediate success!

For others, improvement can be more fleeting. When results become stagnant, I'm simply saying it's okay to step in and play a bigger role in your own recovery. The aim of this book is to help you do just that.

The good news is; illness presents us with an opportunity to see what's important in this life. It does so by sweeping aside the superficial with cold, clinical precision. When we look at life through the lens of serious illness, what we see will either shape us or break us in a heartbeat.

Make no mistake, serious illness is an obnoxious intruder. Keeping it at bay depends largely on your perception of the problem and your desire to overcome it. *Let's explore this a little.*

All illness brings with it two burning questions: what do I have, and how is it treatable?

While these types of questions are justifiable, they can also be thought of as looking at the outer layers of an onion. To penetrate the center of the onion we need to ask ourselves a more probing question: *why did I become ill?* Once we have the why, the what and the how all begin to fall neatly into line.

How do I know this?

I've been seriously ill and lived to tell the tale. I also found the medical profession unable to cope with the complexity of my symptoms. But with a persistent nature and a diligent mind, I succeeded in reclaiming my health after educated people had failed me. Had I known back then what I know now, I could have avoided my illness altogether!

My findings are presented here as a coherent roadmap, leading you to a place of wellness. You can think of the following chapters as missing pieces of a puzzle. Depending on your situation, you may need some of them, or you may need them all.

It should come as no surprise many of these findings run contrary to what is embraced by mainstream medicine. They will also fly in the face of what you now believe to be true. They have to or your health would already be thriving.

When the body is in a full-blown crisis there is no room for middle ground. The gold standard for finding what works should be simple and unassuming. Something either works or it does not.

From this point forward, your health is free to go in any direction that brings positive results. But there are no shortcuts; it takes an effort to become unwell and an equal effort to pull away from it. With that in mind, it's important not to skip over any sections in this book. I strongly urge you to also take full advantage of the video links being offered along the way.

So, shall we begin?

Our miraculous arrival in this life is celebrated with cake; our departure is more difficult to comprehend. When faced with the option of cake or death, we assure ourselves that 80+ years is somehow owed to us, preferring to think of illness as the *other* person's disease.
I hate to be the one to break this disheartening news so early on, but that body you live in has an expiration date. There comes a day when we all

turn to dust. **How we get there, and when, is defined by the choices we make today.**

It's a little harsh, I know, but the importance of health begins to shift the moment it registers that serious illness already knows your name. Like a visitor that's coming but you aren't sure when, illness has little regard for whom it calls on. It flirts with black and white, young and old, and even makes a fool of the rich man. With patient curiosity, illness waits for even the busiest of people in the cruel hope of one day stopping them dead in their tracks.

Often times, we allow life to become a cozy loop of polite conversation and shopping excursions. All sprinkled with an incalculable number of hours watching mind-numbing television. It's all a fleeting distraction that serious illness wipes away with ease.

Very few people on their deathbeds wish they had spent more time reading the Facebook posts of complete strangers. So it seems illness can actually be a beautiful gift. For it is here, in the midst of adversity that we find out what's important and who we really are.

And while it's true, a visit from illness can teach us much, serious illness has the power to consume. Trust me, having walked through the valley of death once, I wouldn't wish it on my worst enemy.

Friend, heed this warning: an ounce of prevention will always outperform a pound of cure. We are all offered the same choice: make time for health now or take time out for sickness later.

FIRST FIND THE WHY

It's worth remembering that illness rarely falls from the deep blue sky— there *has* to be a reason—the trick is to find what's stressing the body and then develop a strategy to overcome it. Along the way, our symptoms can serve as important clues. Some symptoms are subtle; others are more pronounced. *All are relevant.*

Clues may come as profuse sweating or debilitating migraines. Others may come as intense itching, unique body odors, intolerable joint pain, and even a silent hankering for sanity.

And here's the rub ...

The medical system is quick to tell you your suffering is merely genetic, bad luck, or simply old age. When blame is neatly nudged in your direction, a feeling of helplessness ensues. This damning news presents a much bigger problem for you than it does to the doctor treating you.

For now, let's agree to suspend such wasteful thoughts. **If one other person has successfully dealt with the health issue you face, then there are no–as in zero–good reasons why you can't overcome it too.** Your body is a complex marvel with an innate ability to heal itself. Sometimes, we just need to get out of the way and allow it.

All too often we allow ourselves to become conditioned that ill health is somehow inevitable, rather than making a conscious effort to improve it. A few misplaced words from a well-meaning specialist can leave a person feeling like a rudderless ship left to drift on open water. But it doesn't have to be this way; all health problems have solutions, the same as all doors have keys.

HERE'S THE HOW

The path to restoring good health should always be clear and uncomplicated. Toxins must come out of the body and clean nutrients must flow in. Put simply, give your body what it needs and steer it well away from what it doesn't. To help you do this, all of the information you need is in the palm of your hand.

Moving forward, we'll discuss how to keep toxic substances out of your home and your workspace. And by the end of this book, you will also know what to eat and when to eat it without ever getting overwhelmed or confused.

But first, I'd like to share with you a little of my own story. It gets a little ugly at times but there is a certain beauty to any catalyst that brings about permanent change.

HITTING A BRICK WALL

Serious illness is a highly effective teacher, always bringing into focus what is important. For me, it also felt like I'd hit a brick wall at 100 mph. The world I suddenly entered became a place of frustration, fear, and uncompromising pain – hence going back there is no longer an option for me. *Now I listen, now I hear.*

What I found to be true is that the majority of health problems *aren't* lacking in solutions. Rather, in this technological age, there can be too much information to choose from. Fortunately, I'm offering you a way to blast through that mass of digital information. This becomes the fast-track to a less stressed, more energized, healthier version of you!

The following chapter explains how I became deathly ill and why this book was written. Before we jump in, I'd again like to point out this is not a path for those who have yet to give traditional medicine a chance to succeed. Nor is it a good fit for those who are firm in the belief that mainstream medicine will always prevail. But for those who have tried the conventional route and have become frustrated by a lack of progress, then this book is for you –Enjoy!

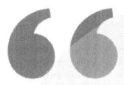

Come if you must with an open mind,

or do not come at all.

Only then will you find value.

– James Lilley

Chapter 2

THE TURNING OF A TOXIC WORM

This is not some elaborate program that you need to buy into. I have no expensive pills or products to sell you. The absence of product links in this book is intentional. From this point on my affiliation is with you alone.

I am keenly aware that this is a book about your health and I have that task firmly in my mind. However, before we set off on this journey together, I'd like to take this opportunity to introduce myself. The aim of retelling my story is pure and simple. It's to convey a clear message that I get it. Illness can be devastating, but somehow, I learned to navigate my own way out of it.

It's debatable what the best way to learn is. Some could argue that first-hand experience is most effective; others will argue for formal learning. While both styles have merit, seeking answers out of pure necessity, is a little different than learning as part of a lucrative career choice.

Example: ask any qualified veterinarian about the strength of a pit bull's jaw and you are sure to get a detailed reply. But if you want to know how sharp the dog's teeth are, find a mailman who's been bitten by one. When you live it, you'd better understand it. Real life experience has a value—more so when your health depends on it, as mine did.

> Experience without theory is blind, but theory without experience is mere intellectual play. –Immanuel Kant

All the techniques I used in my own recovery are inside this book. If you are in a rush to get well, feel free to skip these next few chapters and I'll meet you at the beginning of chapter five. But if you are curious to know how serious illness affected me personally, then keep reading. This is the preferred route and it doesn't take long to read.

Our story begins in the north of England where it seems my life has always moved in units of five. Leaving school at the age of fifteen, it's fair to say I had learned how to write and fight. The relevance of this will become more obvious in later chapters.

Throughout my teenage years, life wasn't always easy but for some reason, my dad never lost faith in me. A man of great patience, he also gave me my gift of unbending persistence. Little did I know this quality would one day save my life.

A five-year stint in the British military gave me a chance to straighten out. The local paper ran a story on me as I won an award for physical training. Fast-forward to the end of my military career and I found myself right back where I started, moving with ease in a tough neighborhood.

Against all odds, I again managed to break free of my stale environment. For the next five years, I ran a successful business with almost fifty employees, and in doing so my life went from rags to riches. That time, the local radio station came.

Zip forward five more years and the breakup of a long-term relationship found me alone and without a business. I felt I needed to get away and found myself standing on American soil. This is where it gets interesting.

HERE SHE COMES

When I arrived in the United States I stumbled upon an unusual ally. In a crowded bar she caught me looking and, when a smile came back, it lit up the room. With a face that wouldn't have been out of place on the cover of a magazine, her natural beauty quickly drew me in.

She was elegant and had a warm, intelligent voice. As most Americans do, she enjoyed listening to my heavy British accent, curious opinions, and even my terrible jokes. I mentioned she looked exactly like my second wife. Her eyes widened and she asked me how many wives I'd had?

Without missing a beat, I said, "Just one."

She must have found me as charming as I was trying to be because one year later she really did become my second wife. We decided to move out of the city and found ourselves embracing a much simpler lifestyle than either of us had been accustomed to. Deep in the heart of rural America, we purchased an old farmhouse in need of repair; this was to be our American dream.

That summer I worked my butt off. If I wasn't busy fixing something inside, I'd be up on the roof or down in the basement crawling around doing some type of repair. I'd always liked solving problems by working them backward and then re-applying common sense and logic to them. It never occurred to me that one day this type of thinking would help me out of a wheelchair.

My beautiful wife had long suspected that I was a workaholic. For me, peace came from working with a purpose. I actually enjoyed being outside in the rain chopping firewood in preparation for a long winter ahead. My parents had been hard workers and a strong work ethic had been instilled in me from an early age. I guess I was fortunate to have inherited an intuitive mind and a surplus of energy, seven days a week.

Several happy years of married life breezed past and we remained inseparable best friends. By now I was submerged in the local lifestyle and grateful to have found a corner of the world very different from the one I grew up in. Living in a small mountain community gave me the opportunity to see that doing the right thing was more important than doing the easy thing.

Here, it was refreshing to find a man's word still had value. I became a product of my new environment and it turned me into an honest and dedicated family man. Together, my wife and I raised a small family and grew a garden. Life was good. Up until that point in my life, serious illness was a stranger to me.

AND HERE "IT" COMES

I'd always been one of the lucky ones; as a child, I once got chicken pox but bounced right back within a week or so. I'd perhaps get a cold every

27

other year but before you could say "sick note" I'd be over it and back at work. In short, my immune system was working just as it was intended.

But, by the beginning of 2011 things were about to change beyond anything I could have foreseen or comprehended. A routine visit to a health center found me sitting in front of a female doctor who encouraged me to be proactive with my health.

At 10:15 a.m. on the 16th of February she suggested I protect myself from a list of diseases that, honestly, had never been much of a problem to me. But like most people, I wanted to do the right thing, and following through with my doctor's advice seemed like the right thing to do. By 10:30 that morning, the ink on my consent form was dry and I'd put my full trust in the medical establishment. By doing so, I had also handed over complete responsibility for my health. And this is where it gets tricky. *Here's why.*

What had just happened to me is an area of medicine that has become the source of many heated discussions. Some folks are for it and some folks are against it. It doesn't matter to me which group you are in, only that you understand **this wasn't my fault.** I simply did what the good doctor suggested, and for whatever reason, things went wrong. If it makes you more comfortable, most people seem to do just fine with this procedure. Me? I'm about to become a statistic. And although this wasn't my fault, it was now my problem.

Beyond that, I'm going to respectfully refrain from going into more detail. At this early stage in the book, I'm not looking to put myself in the center of a polarizing debate. Please note, this story has no hidden agenda. This isn't about being pro or anti anything, I'm simply explaining how things unfolded.

So, shall we just press on?

As I left the health center something didn't quite feel right. I'd never been seriously ill in my life so I shook it off, confident whatever had just happened would work itself out, as it always had.

By the time I got home a few things already felt different. My neck was ultra-tight as if I had somehow pulled a muscle, and both hamstrings were in a state of tension. By nightfall, my head was pounding and I was sensing the beginning of an illness I hadn't experienced before.

Over the next few days, my body alternated between burning up and shivering violently in a sweat-drenched bed. My teeth actually chattered on occasion and a feeling of uneasiness washed over me. As each new morning broke, I found myself already awake and staring at the ceiling.

Unfortunately, I still had work left to do and I was determined to finish it so I could go back to bed in peace. While picking up my car keys to leave the house it felt as if I'd put a large stone in my pocket. I'd never noticed the weight of a key before, so that was a little strange. As I got into my pickup truck, I clipped the top of my head on the doorframe and then did the exact same thing again when I got out. *What the...?*

I'd only climbed back out of the vehicle to check the deck for lost fluid because, on that day of all days, the power steering fluid seemed to have sprung a leak. As I scanned the ground for leaked fluid, I felt my shoulders and head drop simultaneously. The dry ground underneath the truck told me that the fault wasn't with the power steering; it was with my arms.

These were arms used to hard work. They often toiled from sun up to sun down and yet here I was struggling to turn the damned steering wheel on my pickup truck.

As the morning progressed I forced myself to keep moving. I've always prided myself on finishing anything I start but by midday, lifting everyday objects became too much. I settled for dragging them, and myself, around. By lunchtime, my body was under siege and I needed to go home.

PIN?

This is where things started to get even more bizarre. When I stopped for gas, I couldn't remember my debit card PIN number. The bank later called to say I had left my card in the ATM machine. I'd **always** been diligent with money so this was an absolute first for me. Once home, the slightest noise became an irritation. It got to the point where I couldn't even think straight. The tick-tick-ticking clock, a ball bouncing outside, the sound of water running; all seemed to be magnified.

Then my eyes began to bother me, giving way to a sharp, intense pain, which seemed to come and go at random, particularly in my right eye. Both eyes developed ultra-sensitivity to light and, as nightfall came around again, I lay in the dark awake and alone with my thoughts.

Usually, around bedtime, my wife and I would smile and say goodnight to each other to signal the end of each long day. Under the circumstances, I did my best, but tonight it wasn't my usual smile and it was clear I hadn't even come close to fooling her.

As the weeks progressed, so too did my symptoms. My sleep was impaired by harrowing nightmares that leached into my mind with horrific regularity. It felt as if the gates of hell had slammed shut behind me. What worries me to this day is I didn't even see this coming.

But it was my legs that were now my biggest concern. I'd always carried a spring in my step – these were legs that enjoyed walking; now they felt different. Gripped in a constant state of tension. This feeling was most evident in both hamstrings, even as I lay in bed.

As I tried to make sense of what was happening to me, a torrent of questions flooded my mind. Answers did not. Was it the muscles in my legs or could it be the tendons or maybe even the nerves? But if this was a form of neuropathy, was it myopathy or polyneuropathy? Could this be the start of some new autoimmune condition that had been primed to attack from within? Or was it ALS or MS? Around and around and around in endless circles with no answer to be found.

The only thing I knew for sure was my previously robust immune system had been compromised. And these alarming sensations weren't leaving my side. As someone who likes to be productive, I hated being sick. Days soon began to melt into nights with annoying repetition. After another week of incessant illness, my biggest fear was I wasn't bouncing back.

Up until this point in my life, I had rarely seen a doctor, nor had my elderly parents. It had been a successful strategy that had allowed my health to flourish unhindered; now I was paying the price for allowing others to meddle.

I hated the very thought of going back to the doctor with every fiber in my body. I was actually relieved when the receptionist announced in an upbeat tone, "It will be another week before we can get you back in again."

Each new day presented more problems with no end in sight. I watched in absolute horror as random muscles now began to twitch throughout my body. This unsettled me and, deep down, I knew I was in trouble.

A string of futile doctor visits soon began to be the only thing worth dragging myself out of bed for. If anyone had the elusive answers I needed, they weren't telling.

Throughout this period my elderly parents began telephoning every day from England to check in on me. Dad would try to cheer me up with his brand of terrible jokes. (Why do dads do that?) Mom wasn't quite so upbeat; it was clear from the crackled tone in her voice she was suffering right along with me. I can only imagine what she was thinking as her only son lay on a sickbed in a faraway land alternating between hardship and pain.

As time edged forward I could sense we were already at the back end of winter and spring was approaching. I desperately wanted to be working outside in the cool spring air as I always had, but by the time spring ended I had spent most of it confined to my bedroom. There had been several nights when it felt as if the coldness of death wanted to climb deep inside me. And there were a few times I wished it had.

Going to the doctors now became my only outdoor activity. It was of little comfort my blood tests had all come back as "normal." The irony

31

was the doctor who propelled me into this shitty mess was now the same one trying to get me out of it.

Her advice to be "proactive" with my health had spectacularly backfired. Unable to figure out what had gone wrong, she then referred me to another doctor, and then another. Maybe you can relate?

Now too weak to work, I again took to my sweat-drenched bed and prayed for this all to go away. Being the independent problem-solving type, I'd spent most of my adult life being self-employed and I liked it that way. But I was now in the undesirable position of being too ill to work, but not quite ill enough to die.

Without any type of safety net, another month or so passed. But for my wife and I, the marking of time wasn't passing so easy. Without a paycheck coming in we were now slipping into financial decline. The absurdity of the situation was that, even in the grip of serious illness, I still wanted to do the right thing and pay my bills on time. Quietly, one by one, the things I had worked so hard for all began creeping out the door.

Despite the hardship that comes from choosing to live a life in rural America, there is also a strong sense of community—more so in the mountains. As our situation continued to go from bad to worse, the news of what was happening to our family trickled through the small, tight-knit community.

Get Well Soon cards began to appear in our mailbox with prepaid grocery cards tucked inside them. Another envelope came with no note, just a $100 bill inside. These were not people of any great wealth, but they were people who pressed hard cash into the hand of anyone in need and refused to accept no for an answer.

As a fiercely independent person, it's never been easy for me to accept help from anyone. A month later I reluctantly sold my pickup truck. Fortunately, we still had my wife's car as a backup. Being driven to and from doctors' appointments by my wife soon had me floundering in my own self-pity.

This is where unhelpful male pride begins to kick in. I remember thinking this isn't how I live; this isn't who I am. I know, right? A prideful heart that needs to be taught humility; unfortunately, this harsh lesson was only just beginning.

To help keep us afloat, my wife turned her hand to selling knitting patterns online. How she managed to remain creative under this level of stress is beyond me. Thankfully, a small flurry of sales always seemed to come in when we needed them the most. I was thankful we shared a modest two-bedroom house with small bills. Had it not been for these combining factors I doubt we would have been able to keep the lights on.

OLD SCHOOL

At this point, you may be wondering why I didn't try to sue the doctor who had sent me into this unintended tailspin. This is America; everyone sues in America, right? First, you have to understand I was ill, and doing the best I could to get through each terrifying day. Also, when you discover you are the one standing at the edge of the abyss, the last thing on your mind is fighting over money in court.

I'm also old school: the whole suing culture thing has never sat right with me. I didn't want to spend my days hanging on for handouts. I wanted to get well and get back to work. What good would it do me anyway? I still didn't have a current diagnosis and, before entering into this mess, I'd been handed that medical disclaimer to sign. It seemed that, in the event of something going wrong, the doctor's back was covered. But mine? Meh, not so much.

Back home I watched from my bedroom window as spring turned to summer. I could see weeds had taken my once pristine garden hostage, which seemed to mirror what was happening in my ailing body. Downstairs I overheard someone ask, "Hey, why is your grass getting so long?" The world through other people's eyes; you have to love it. My immaculate garden had always been so full of order and pride. Maybe they thought the grass fairy came and did it, who knows?

I had now been seriously ill in bed, alternating between shivering and sweating, for six long months. More doctors' appointments ensued and yet a solution remained as elusive as ever. Such bright doctors trying to unravel a complicated problem without, it seemed, a thread of common sense between them.

Naively, I was still convinced I was about to shake this off any day. But my symptoms continued to ebb and flow with annoying repetition. The only thing to change was the unkempt view from my window. Fall had long been my favorite. This year, watching maple leaves fall to the ground was a little harder to do because it signaled the end of another missed season. Winter was now approaching.

When it snows in the northern mountains of New Hampshire there is no telling when it will stop; that year the snow came early. I needed to be outside plowing the driveway but, through no fault of my own, this was no longer an option.

As I watched the snow quicken, a local contractor pulled into the drive with a rusty yellow plow attached to the front of his truck. Holding his collar to the wind he made his way to the back door. Evidently, he had heard of my plight and offered to plow the drive in exchange for hot coffee. With every spare penny being counted, this was one less thing to worry about.

As things continued to go from bad to worse, the thought of Christmas coming filled me with dread. This was the first time I'd been unable to provide for my family and it was proving difficult to accept. A new question began to churn in my brain like a toxic worm—*what use am I if I can't even provide for my own family at Christmas?*

Leaving behind only silent footprints in the snow, someone stepped in and donated a large bag of Christmas presents. The accompanying card simply read "Merry Christmas." While this anonymous act of kindness was appreciated, it was also deeply humbling. With a streak of stubborn independence still running through me, I always felt more at ease struggling than accepting offers of help. I was now finding a new awkwardness in accepting that which I had not worked for. The brick wall I was hitting took hold of my ridiculous male pride and began to shred it.

I'd been standing on my own two feet from a very early age. But now my claims that I'd never needed help from anyone became irrelevant background noise. Life was teaching me some pretty harsh lessons. Perhaps the gods had noticed my longing for self-reliance and mistaken it for defiance. Either way, illness was about to bring me to my knees, and I wasn't in any position to argue.

As the rest of the festive world continued to turn with selfish repetition, the strain on my beautiful wife's face was becoming plain to see. Worry had replaced optimism and her once raven black hair now displayed streaks of pure grey. This wasn't an easy time for either of us and, at times, it showed more than we would have liked. The next morning, seeing her brown leather suitcase on the bed made me wonder if things could get any worse.

I wasn't going to beg her to stay, for begging is not my prideful business. I guess turning to say goodbye was too much emotion for one day. Still visibly upset from an earlier argument, she wiped away a fresh tear and put the suitcase away. It was obvious we still cared about each other the way only families can.

No matter what life was throwing at us, we were still inseparable best friends. From this point forward, it was clear we were in this together.

As Christmas 2011 ended, it also brought with it a naïve glimmer of hope. A new year was looming and we both longed to put the current heinous one behind us. What we didn't know was that things were about to take a dramatic turn for the worse.

Chapter 3

DEATH BY 1000 PAPER CUTS

January 2012 brought with it our sixth wedding anniversary. We celebrated the day by visiting a neurologist from a neighboring hospital. I know right, who says romance is dead?

The test carried out that day was to check the nerves in my legs. This was done by sending an electrical pulse down the nerve via a needle. Each turn of the dial caused my leg to twitch involuntarily. At one point, my wife needed to excuse herself from the room. Evidently, she has a warped sense of humor.

The neurologist gently put his hand on my shoulder and encouraged me to relax. This led me to believe at least one of us in the protocol was failing to grasp the fullness of the situation.

Fifteen minutes later the sadist in the white coat declared I could stop "relaxing" as my nerves had passed the test. He then handed me a bill for $530 and sent me on my way. Sheesh, thanks, doc.

> "We cannot solve our problems with the same thinking
> we used when we created them" – Albert Einstein

However helpful this test may have been to the neurologist, it wasn't helpful to me. Adding to the problem, the doctor who had inadvertently set me on this path was still unable to provide answers. It began to bother me that I was being viewed as just another sick guy shuffling from appointment to appointment.

I'm actually a real person. At my core, I was still somebody's son, husband, and brother. It also registered I had now been seriously ill for almost a year. For someone who rarely got sick, this was proving hard to accept.

While I waited for answers, my immune system continued acting up. I'd never had an allergy before in my life! Now watery eyes, sneezing, and itching all became a daily annoyance and nobody seemed willing (or able) to connect the dots.

Over the coming months, things continued downhill. Using a metal walker for the first time made me realize how far my previously robust health had fallen. Adding to my endless list of problems, I now found myself needing to use the bathroom every five minutes making rest impossible.

I really needed this symptom like a hole in the head. Being forced to scramble to the toilet all night long soon became stressful. For a while, when you don't have a choice, you learn to adapt. My latest coping strategy was to sleep a few minutes at a time. Sometimes I did this with my forehead on the toilet roll holder. At some point, I went back to the doctor and begged for a solution. She ordered a series of urine tests. Go figure–they all came back normal.

With some degree of desperation, I went home and did my best to cope. Each night the same pattern repeated. Normal people went to bed while I shuffled from the bedroom to bathroom using a walker. The longer I went without a full night's sleep; the harder life became. It's only a matter of time before something has to give.

A lack of sleep conspired against my every positive thought. Each night I'd walk the darkest corridors of my mind. This was now becoming a regular and unsustainable occurrence.

SICK-NOTE

Also around this time, the doctor whose advice I had taken on February 16th, 2011, sent a letter to my house. It started by stating that she was leaving to take up another job in a different practice. At some point, she used the phrase, "It is with a heavy heart that I am leaving."

It crossed my mind that holding onto furniture as I walked across a room was reason for a heavy heart. Watching my wife struggle to pay for groceries was reason for a heavy heart. But skipping town for a better paying fucking job? No, that was not a reason for a heavy heart. And, given my situation, maybe even a tad insensitive!

I was now being slammed with debilitating fatigue, tightness in my muscles, weak arms, irritability and weak legs. Let's not forget painful eyes, heart palpitations, hot sweats, cold sweats, new food sensitivities, twitching muscles, new seasonal allergies, jaw clenching, confusion, sleep deprivation and ongoing horrific nightmares. All matched by an equally worrisome fresh crop of fatty lipomas that had begun to spring up all over my body. Oh, and just for good measure, around the clock trips to the bathroom.

As a previously active person, I was horrified at the thought of losing my independence. It's a little unnerving when you live with good health for most of your life and then your legs become strangely tight for more than a year. It was incomprehensible to think of one day being trapped in a wheelchair, but by that time it was no longer a question of if, but rather when.

UNSUSTAINABLE

It's very easy to judge someone from the sidelines. But sooner or later the stress of prolonged fatigue will bring you to a breaking point. The feeling of letting everyone down was becoming unsustainable. I know what you are thinking because I thought it too: if this problem is no longer sustainable then how can it be stopped?

As problems go, this one caused me considerable anguish. As the night air cooled, it eventually gained a mathematical probability. Determined to spare someone the inconvenience of cleaning up my mess, I found myself outside, kneeling before God with an open heart and a loaded gun. A sure sign that a previously robust man was now on the edge.

Trembling like a pathetic wet dog, the fear of the unknown finally gave way to a sweaty but insistent right hand. Without further distraction, a single round went into the chamber and from here, it doesn't get more real. As if it even mattered, I glanced at my watch and, at 4:22 a.m., I finally lost all hope.

The first of two cold metallic snaps went off next to the right side of my head – which then echoed away endlessly into the blackness of the night. The deafening silence that followed was interrupted by a pounding heart fueled by a steady supply of fresh adrenaline.

If nothing else was going right for me then at least math appeared to be on my side. When you reach this point of desperation, the only question to cross a tormented mind is this: why am I being forced to endure this nightmare?

Either way, enduring it seemed like the better choice. And at that moment, that's what I was determined to do. By this time, the doctor who had lit the fuse to my health problems had moved on with her heavy heart to a better paying job. So I met with several new "specialists" to review my medical records. Two of them were nice and one was actually quite arrogant. None completely understood the complexity of what was happening to me.

Suppressing symptoms is what doctors do best and I was offered drugs to pacify me. But I wasn't looking for easy painkillers to mask symptoms; I wanted a solution. To me, at least, this type of thinking is no different from a fireman climbing into a burning house only to cut the wire to the smoke detector. The twisted logic of no alarm = no problem tends to work best when it's not your house that's burning.

During each visit to the doctors, my wife stood firmly by my side and, with great dignity, we thanked each doctor for their time. She would then help me up out of my seat and through the door. The day my wife took the initiative and brought home a used wheelchair from a charity shop was one of the lowest moments of my life. Even now, as I write this several years later, that day still makes me choke up.

I remember being annoyed she even brought it to the house. Stubbornness told me I didn't need it, but in truth, I'd needed it some time ago. I was afraid if my beautiful wife saw me sitting in it she might begin to see only the chair. It also crossed my mind that once I sat down I might never get up again. To be clear, I hadn't lost the use of my legs, it had simply reached the point where using them was too slow and too painful.

Reluctantly I handed over my walker and took my first seat in this damned ugly-looking metal contraption. Admitting defeat wasn't something I took lightly but by now my self-worth had begun to drip out from under me. I felt humiliated as if I had given up.

It's not until you sit in a wheelchair that you begin to see the world from a very difficult perspective—literally. It might not look it, but getting a wheelchair to move is cumbersome and hard work on the arms, especially when you don't feel well, to begin with.

I must have complained about it because a week later my mother-in-law drove 223 miles to deliver an electric wheelchair. Like her, it had a few miles on it, but I'm guessing it still must have cost her a small fortune. And there I was, slouched deep in an electric wheelchair and needing a moment to be alone.

The irony is, the procedure I got myself roped into back in February 2011 was supposed to provide immunity against disease. I was told it was "safe and effective" with zero mention of a downside.

Mainstream medicine, with all its sophistication, had failed me. I was now just another little guy slipping through the medical cracks.

Even science with its pristine reputation for accuracy was sulking in the corner, wondering if Pluto was a planet or not.

NEW DOCTORS

Waiting for someone else to figure out my health problems had been the plan for two long years. A new doctor then arrives on the scene. I soon found that when a new doctor doesn't have the time or experience to figure out complex health problems, conceit takes precedence over common sense. Especially when faced with a problem (that's you) that won't go away or, doesn't fit into any typical example or pattern,

If we aren't careful, the onus of blame is conveniently shifted onto the patient. This ensures that, at the end of each shift, messy problems fit into neat little boxes. Do you see what's going on here?

 The doctor is basically saying "Hey, I don't actually understand your complicated symptoms but I'm paid to be smart, so it can't possibly be me. So, for now, let's say you are the problem!"

This repulsively flawed logic only serves to protect the ego of an ignorant person who lacks facts. The sheer arrogance of any doctor to make this distasteful suggestion was sure to be the last.

I wasn't to blame, hell no! I had done everything asked of me. Back in 2011, it hadn't been my brilliant idea to provoke my immune system into a total meltdown.

I'd since turned up for every appointment and sat quietly and respectfully while being prodded and poked. I'd be damned if I was now going to allow someone to add insult to my injury. I hadn't brought this on myself in any way, shape or form. Enough of this horse shit. I was done!

Whatever it took, whatever I had to sacrifice, whatever I had to learn, I was determined to do it or drop dead trying. My dad used to say, "A determined man will always find a way; a lesser man will find an excuse."

I was done having my destiny be controlled by the ignorance of others. I certainly wasn't going to sit back and subject myself to more of this nonsense. Now I was ready to roll up my sleeves and fight in my own corner and boy did I have a point to make!

> Survival was my only hope, success my only revenge.
> – Patricia Cornwell.

When the human spirit hits the right motivational spot it has an uncanny ability to triumph over adversity. History books are full of persistent people who refuse to be told something can't be done.

Remember those two bicycle repairmen who once asked the question, "If a bird can fly, why can't man?" Aviation, as we know it today, came as a direct result of the Wright brothers' persistence. But I wasn't looking to fly; I only needed to walk.

Let's take stock of what I had going for me, (a) I had a point to prove, (b) I'm persistent, (c) I was still of this world and (d) I had a wife that needed me. For most people that will do it.

Every night while the rest of the town slept, I began the slow and laborious process of figuring out what had gone wrong. Today I walk unaided and sleep through the night. My mind is at peace and I have the energy to be able to work on demand. Yes, a few stubborn quirks remain but 95% of my original symptoms are now under my control. Given the severity of my earlier condition, I regard this as a remarkable success.

Here's how I did it.

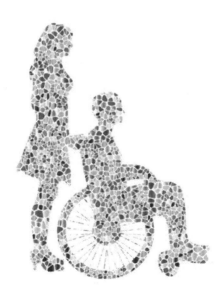

Chapter 4

INFINITE POSSIBILITIES

When faced with a long list of complicated problems, knowing where to begin becomes key. Sadly, this pivotal piece of information eluded me and several years of failure followed. But giving up wasn't something I do readily or particularly well.

My wife has often referred to me as being the most persistent man she has ever met; to me, each defeat became a new learning experience. This gave me a defining and favorable edge over most of my doctors who—I was quick to notice—all went home at 5 p.m.

Clearly, there was only going to be one eventual outcome; how long it would take to get there was a different matter. I also knew my own body better than anyone else, and I'm guessing you know yours too. If anything, it helps to have a little more skin in the game.

> If you can read, you can learn everything that anyone ever learned, but you've got to want it. – Ricky Gervais

A realization hit me that schools and doctors were no longer the ultimate gatekeepers of all knowledge. Every day people learn new skills online from building a boat to baking a cake. It's all right there in the public domain.

For anyone with a burning desire to learn, Dr. Google is a tool of infinite possibilities. I soon found academics, physicians, and professors all sharing information right there on my desktop. The problem I now faced wasn't a lack of information but how to filter out so much of it.

BENCHMARK

Rather than let it consume me, I devised a plan to refine my search. I figured if someone held a Ph.D., they had to have a certain level of credibility. This was my new benchmark and these were the minds I would seek first. I then discovered TedTalks.com, which gave me a way to tap into some of the brightest minds from around the world.

I became completely submerged in the task ahead of me, losing all track of time. Birthdays came and went, as did the 4th of July, Christmas, and the Super Bowl. Days, nights, weekends and cookouts all passed me by as I sucked information from anybody that had it.

Everything else became a distraction. Finding the answer wasn't just something I needed to do; it had become an insatiable passion.

You need a lot of passion for what you're doing because it's so hard. Without passion, any rational person would give up. – Steve Jobs.

My appetite for medical knowledge knew no bounds. I'd read while sitting in the bathtub and I'd read on every car ride as my wife drove along, talking to herself. It's funny how we dislike being taught and yet, when something is important to us, we have an unquenchable thirst to learn.

It wasn't uncommon for me to be fact-checking long before my wife woke up and long after she had gone to bed. With no one paying for my web-ucation my only goal was to press on and find something that worked. Yet, despite all these efforts, so much of my own puzzle remained elusive.

In a bid to find the missing pieces, I began to cross-reference what I had already learned. In doing so, a rich vein of insight opened up that, until then, hadn't even been on my radar.

There were other people who were also suffering and keen to share their experiences. Health forums are full of regular people just like you and me. Some are there searching for answers; others are there to share their successes.

On the one hand, I was becoming well read from PhDs, and on the other hand, I now had access to people with valuable firsthand experience.

Piece by piece I was beginning to get a grasp of the scope of the problem.

The task ahead remained both tantalizing and daunting, but for the first time, I felt there was light at the end of a hideously dark tunnel. I began putting the small things I had learned into practice. As with so many other persistent people before me, my progress was often sidelined by a spectacular, but short-lived, failure. But as time went on, even the smallest of victories empowered me.

I began to enjoy a slow but steady improvement in my symptoms. I was now moving around on a cane and doing so with a huge smile on my face because I was having success where my doctors had not.

So how does a layperson find his or her way out of a medical maze? That same word keeps coming back: persistence. Had this trait not been instilled in me from a very early age I wouldn't be writing this. My dad had always admired this characteristic more than any other. He often said things like, "People are free to mock the man that tries, but they should never underestimate him."

Today, as I write with enthusiasm, I have seen a 95% improvement in my original symptoms. Quite remarkably I managed to do this while taking zero medications. The majority of my symptoms are reduced to the point where they no longer control me: I control them.

Had I known in 2011, what I know now, I could have averted my illness altogether. At the very least my recovery would have happened much sooner.

Up until this point writing about my past hasn't been easy but, with the stage now set, my writing shackles can finally come off!

My new challenge is to take these fundamental concepts and convey them in a way without it sounding like mundane, medical mantra. This is what excites me. Come, we have much work to do.

Chapter 5

YOU DON'T HAVE AN ILLNESS, YOU HAVE A LABEL

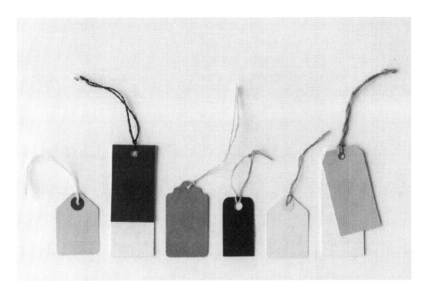

In its most basic form, every living thing on this planet is made up of cells. From plants to animals, from trees to humans, wherever there is life there are cells. If we look under a microscope, you and I are little more than a mass of cells tightly wrapped in a layer of skin.

Just as a house is made of thousands of bricks, trillions of these tiny cells make up your eyes, lungs, brain, fingers, nose, and toes. Cells also make up just about every other bit of yourself you can think of. Essentially, cells are the building blocks of all this life and the smallest living unit that can replicate independently.

What's the relevance of knowing that you and I are home to trillions of microscopic cells?

Think about it … if we are to accurately manage what ails us, our first goal must be to break down the complex into something more manageable. Looking at a problem in its most basic form (the cell) allows us to develop a fresh perspective of illness. To some, what you are about to read may seem like an oversimplification, but this is just our base which we will then build on as each chapter unfolds.

> If you can't explain it simply, you don't understand it well enough. — Albert Einstein.

As you read this paragraph, your old worn out cells are being replaced. This turnover forms an essential cycle of life. We could think of this process as deleting unwanted photos from our cell phone; once that space is freed up, the system works better.

KEEP, KILL, OR RECYCLE?

To make way for healthy new cells your body makes a judgment call to either keep, kill, or recycle damaged cells. When cells are recycled, the body eats them, a process known as autophagy. This term stems from the Greek word, "self-devouring."

When a cell is deemed damaged beyond repair it's encouraged to commit suicide, a process often referred to as apoptosis. Under normal circumstances, cells do this in a tightly regulated fashion. When old cells "forget" to commit suicide, problems begin.

If we assume that a healthy organ is made up of mostly healthy cells, we could also assume that an unhealthy organ has at least some unhealthy cells. What we are doing here is breaking the problem down to its most basic form. If the illness is reflected in the structure of our cells, then this is true for just about any illness from A to Z.

Cancer is the most obvious example of an overzealous set of cells malfunctioning beyond the body's ability to regulate them. A diagnosis of cancer can be alarming enough, but if we look a little closer at the problem, the bigger issue always happening at the cellular level. The term cellular is simply a word relating to the cells. The more health issues you have, the more relevant simplification becomes.

Let's look at it another way: a basic four-digit PIN is all we need to provide financial peace of mind. This concept works because the number of combinations is too great to hack. Now imagine trying to unlock a health problem with several hundred possible causes!

To add to the problem, symptoms often overlap. This overlapping of symptoms makes the diagnostic process all the more difficult to navigate. But by breaking down the problem to the cellular level, we can see it from a totally different perspective.

In every area of the body, we either have a collection of healthy cells or not so healthy cells. When it is the latter, we call it an illness. Now we are off to the races and in with a chance of unraveling the complex.

I know what you are thinking because I thought it too: even if an illness is nothing more than a set of wacky malfunctioning cells, how does this help me?

First, let's replace the how question with a why question. When we ask the how question we are surface skimming. But when we ask the "why" question we are forced to dig below the surface for answers.

WHY?

Asking WHY our cells have turned sickly on us is a smart question to ask and the answer is straightforward. For a cell to form or rebuild it requires key nutrients. It rarely bodes well for a cell to be made up of toxic elements.

When new cells build, they take from whatever nutrients the body has at its disposal. A nutrient can be thought of as any substance that provides nourishment essential for the maintenance of life and growth. The quality of these new cells depends on the quality of the raw materials fueling the body. Think of a carpenter trying to build beautiful furniture with rotten wood.

Quality nutrients build quality cells. These nutrients come to us in the foods we eat; this is the fuel the body runs on, whether it is junk food or superfood. Here we see the birth pangs of problem cells. A lack of key nutrients flowing into the cell will affect the cell's quality and optimal integrity. Are you getting this bit? It's kinda important.

With quality nutrients, cell walls remain permeable. This allows the exchange of oxygen-carrying nutrients to come in, and the free flow of toxins out. Anything of a toxic nature will obstruct this rebuilding process.

When any part of our body becomes ill, something is either missing in our healthy cells or it has been replaced by something toxic. In short, we are trying to build a house with substandard bricks and rotten wood.

I'm using the word "toxic" here in its broadest possible sense. Indiscriminately, it could be used to describe any pathogen or foreign matter that has the potential to penetrate your cells and make you ill. It could be a virus, fungus, bacteria, pesticide, drug, heavy metal, chemical, liquid, gas fumes, contaminated food etc.

The list of potential (known) toxic substances is impossibly long. We will, of course, be looking at many of these toxins in more detail along with effective ways to remove them from the body. For the sake of simplicity, we can also think of the word toxic as any substance poisonous to the body.

The body (that's you) is aptly designed to filter out such toxic substances and it does so in a highly efficient fashion. Problems arise when more toxins flood into the body than the body is capable of removing. Unfortunately, humans in our pursuit of progress, have become highly destructive creatures. As a species, we humans are hell-bent on contaminating the world we live in.

Today it has become impossible to avoid dangerous levels of toxicity, hence, awareness becomes key. As a rule of thumb, if you have a pulse then you have some degree of toxicity in your body. Anything that's manmade almost certainly has a toxic element to it.
The good news is, the next chapter covers this in more detail.

It doesn't matter what your doctor calls it, it ALWAYS involves toxicity
— Dr. Sherry Rogers

The body relies on the liver, kidneys, lungs and skin to filter out harmful toxins. In fact, our entire health hinges on the ability of these organs to cope. Once these vital organs begin working overtime, it's easy for the whole system to become overrun. A tipping point usually occurs when the prolonged demand remains too great for the body.

DRIP, DRIP, DRIP

Imagine a bucket catching water drips from a ceiling. As long as the drip is slow the bucket takes a long time to fill up. If the bucket has a slight leak, then one drop in, one drop out maintains a steady level.

In this analogy, think of the drips coming into the bucket as your daily exposure to toxins. And the leak as your detoxification organs working to keep the bucket from filling up.

If the drip coming from the ceiling begins to speed up the water level in the bucket will rise. When the water level reaches the rim, we could think of ourselves on the edge of illness, or at the "tipping point." When the water spills over the sides of the bucket, it's a sign that your body can no longer cope with the demand being put on it.

Life is good when we prevent toxins from building up. We don't want to get to the point where they overtake our detoxification capabilities. The good news is; this book will help you reduce your toxic exposure as well as showing you how to get clean nutrients into your cells. Once the cells get fired up, good things happen!

That said, there is no point in bringing nourishment to a toxic cell. That would be no different than putting a fresh Band-Aid on a cut before washing it. Common sense would suggest that our first goal must be to reduce the number of new toxins coming into the body. At least until the gravity of the situation is assessed.

53

If repetition is the mother of all learning, let's quickly remind ourselves that new cells replace old, worn out cells. These new cells are made from the raw materials that we provide from the things we eat, whether it be carrots, cucumbers or cake. A cell with a toxic element to it is not a healthy cell and illness ensues.

LABELS

Having an illness can make it seem as if our world is coming to an end. Going into a hospital can be a daunting experience, and trying to make sense of it all can drive a person to despair. As a patient, you will be dealing with an organization well versed in terminology that may be unfamiliar to you.

Once we become ill, the first thing a physician wants to do is give the illness a name. A diagnosis is simply a descriptive term relating to a specific part of the body — that's all. No matter what ails you, I'd like to suggest that you really don't have an illness, what you do have is a label. This label is simply reflecting what is going awry at the cellular level.

A complicated diagnosis can leave a patient feeling helpless. A synchronous diaphragmatic flutter, for example, has a serious ring to it, but most of us know it as a hiccup. And that transient lingual papillitis? That's nothing more than a bump on the tongue. I know right? Who talks like this?

This type of terminology can soon become overwhelming, especially if you aren't feeling well to begin with. The next time a doctor provides you with a complicated diagnosis you could try saying to yourself, "Nope, what I have now is a label." Looking at a diagnosis this way helps to charm the mystery out of complex medical terms.

Osteoporosis, as I'm sure many will already know, is the label given to reflect the condition of certain bones. But even bone is made up of cells. We could just as accurately say that something is going wrong with the cells that make up the bones.

By taking the complex and breaking it down into workable parts we begin to unravel a tangled web of symptoms. An autoimmune condition affecting the cartilage of the joints carries an arthritis label. But once again we know that all cartilage is made of cells. Cancer found in the blood carries the leukemia label, but again blood is made up of cells.

Each and every part of the body has its own label, but regardless of the label that's being applied, something untoward is happening at the cellular level.

The suggestion that cells play such a pivotal role in our health might be a different way of thinking, but that tide may now be turning. How so?

In 2016, the Nobel Prize for medicine was awarded to Yoshinori Ohsumi of Japan for his work on none other than cells.

Ohsumi's discoveries are directly related to the importance of how cells recycle their content. How they break down proteins and non-essential components for energy and destroy invading organisms. I guess another way of saying it is that cells are working out whether to keep, kill or recycle themselves.

What did we learn from this?
A diagnosis is nothing more than a label and it shouldn't define who we are. Complicated problems remain complicated unless we break them down into manageable parts.

Getting toxins out of the body allows nutrients to flood in is the essence of good health.

Homework: Your first assignment is to watch a short TED Talk by Dr. Rangan Chatterjee. It's called, "How to make diseases disappear?"
For my online homies, simply click on the link below.

https://www.youtube.com/watch?v=gaY4m00wXpw

Chapter 6

THE WORLD WE LIVE IN

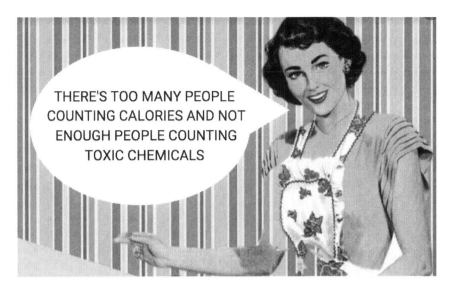

Any substance that has a toxic element to it has the potential to build up in the body. Sometimes this build-up happens quickly; sometimes it happens over time.

Until we make ourselves aware of them, toxins will continue slipping past us with ease. You may choose to ignore these warnings if you wish, but from today it will be difficult to say you weren't aware of them.

So the aim of this chapter is to help you spot potential areas of concern, as well as offering practical solutions. Some of the following information you may be aware of, some of it will shock you to the core!

You may recall how Johnson & Johnson recently paid out millions of dollars for failing to disclose an alleged cancer link to its baby powder! I cannot tell you why some manufacturers think it's okay to put harmful ingredients into our products, but clearly, they do. It's not until we face our own health crisis, that we begin to ask our own questions like "what's making us so sick?"

Supermarkets aren't the ones we can trust to diligently check our products for toxic ingredients. Perhaps it's even a little naive to expect any corporation to police its own income streams.

We have a lot of ground to cover so let's get the ball rolling with the body's largest organ. What we put onto the skin goes into the skin, which in turn gets dumped into the bloodstream. No really, it's true. Especially problematic are oils, cosmetics, bug sprays, creams, perfumes, underarm antiperspirants, yadda, yadda, yadda. If you aren't feeling well, to begin with, these products slowly add to our toxic burden. Drip, drip, drip.

Skin is considered by many to be the body's third kidney. Skin is alive and intelligent. If our goal is to keep illness at bay, then perhaps we should be making life easier for our living, breathing skin.

Still not convinced, huh?

Okay, try this. Every day for the next week try spraying perfume on a houseplant and watch as the leaves begin to curl up and die. Our skin is absorbent in the exact same way.

All too often, we stifle the body's ability to regulate itself. This is achieved by wrapping our skin in layers of manmade fibers. If the shirt you are wearing is made up of the materials below then a rethink may be in order.

Polyester is made from synthetic polymers that come from esters of dihydric alcohol and terpthalic acid. Polyester is perhaps one of the worst fabrics you can wear because it doesn't allow the skin to breathe.

Teflon is increasingly being added to clothing because and the benefit is packaged as wrinkle-free. But most clothing labeled "no-iron" contains carcinogenic PFCs, but don't take my word for it. The U.S. Environmental Protection Agency (EPA) recently announced that PFCs are cancer-causing compounds.

Acrylic fabrics are polycrylonitriles are also known to have carcinogenic qualities.

Rayon is treated with chemicals like caustic soda, ammonia, acetone, and sulphuric acid. All are thought to survive regular washing.

Nylon is made from petroleum and is often given a permanent chemical finish that can irritate the skin.

The goal here isn't to make your life more difficult, it's to first bring awareness to these problems and then offer you viable solutions. So what's the alternative to manmade fibers? That's easy, before manmade materials came along we all used natural fibers like cotton, hemp, or wool. These products remain easy to find and make a good replacement. Natural fibers allow the body to cool without leaching toxic chemicals onto the skin.

Will doing this one thing change your health? I believe the more things you stack in your favor, the better your overall health becomes. On the flip side, we could also say that things of a toxic nature have the potential to compound.

GRAB A PEN AND PAPER

As we now move forward it might be helpful to grab a pen and paper to make a few side notes. There's plenty of solid information coming your way. The good news is, each of the following recommendations is inexpensive and easy to put in place. The much bigger problem is remaining blissfully unaware of them. Without further ado, let's get to it.

SOAP

Anti-bacterial hand soap sounds good but it should be the very first thing you banish to the trash can. Antibacterial soaps contain agents such as triclosan and triclocarban. The dangers of these two agents are many and well documented. They are endocrine disrupters that should have been banned years ago.

Better to use a regular bar of soap like the one Grandma used to use, but even then check the ingredients. The least toxic brands are usually found at your local health food store.

MEDICATIONS

Yup, some medications have life-saving qualities, no question about it. But others may cause a toxic reaction. If your health has become less robust recently then stop what you are doing (even reading this!) and go check the insert.

See if your symptoms match any of the known side effects. If you hit a match, bingo! Talk to your doctor to replace or reduce the dose.

WATER QUALITY

Water is water, right? Meh, not so fast.

Plastic water bottles can leach Bisphenol-A (BPA) into the water. BPA is a synthetic estrogen that can mess up your hormones. Some brands are worse than others, and some are simply filtered tap water. Which begs the question: why not cut out the middleman and install a water filter for your home?

There are lots of filters on the market but ANY filter is better than no filter. I'm not endorsing any product here but Berkey is known to manufacture a range of decent clean water filtration systems. They are simple in design and effective at what they do. That said, Berkey filters aren't the cheapest on the market. But, over time, the cost of buying a good filter is offset by not having to buy plastic water bottles.

If your budget is a little tight, it's better to find a filter that fits your budget today rather than waiting until tomorrow. You can always upgrade later. Without a filter, your kidneys become that filter!

There are tons of water filters out there, but as with most things, you tend to get what you pay for. Reverse osmosis filters are popular because they remove a wide range of impurities. But in doing so they can strip out minerals. You may need to restructure and re-mineralize the water after filtering. This is done by adding minerals back into the water.

Sometimes this can be done automatically during the filtration process. Another way is to allow a jug of filtered water to sit in the fridge overnight, and then add a pinch of Himalayan salt to it. A quick Google search will yield lots more information about how to replace minerals.

If you want to kick this up a notch, you can also test the quality of the water coming into your house. This is easy to do and (compared to illness) relatively inexpensive. Simply call a water specialist firm in your area. They will come out to your home, take a sample, and do the water test for you. If there's a problem (and there usually is) a filter is the answer.

MOLD

Once you have your water checked off the list, the single biggest problem is mold. Mold isn't just the black stuff you see lurking around the bathtub. What I'm referring to here is a much bigger issue and potentially far more dangerous.

Mold can be microscopic and hidden from view. Symptoms can range from brain fog to chronic fatigue. Some people may even express anger or suffer from stubborn weight gain.

Keep an open mind and be aware that some family members are far more sensitive to mold than others. The good news is once you pinpoint a mold problem, life gets a whole lot easier.

The idea here is to become your own detective. Start by asking yourself whether the timing of any health issues corresponded with a house move? Microscopic mold can build up anywhere there is the slightest moisture. Moisture can come from an unseen leaking pipe in the ceiling, wall, or under the floorboards. Be on the lookout for any tell-tale signs such as brown water marks on ceilings.

It pays to be vigilant, water damage can be cleaned up by a landlord. But what lurks beneath carpets and behind sheetrock often goes unseen. If you are unsure, ask your neighbors if your home has flooded in the past.

To help you, there's a test called an ERMI mold test. It's an objective, standardized DNA based method of testing that will identify and quantify molds. At the time of writing, the test costs around $290. But again, think about lost work hours, doctor's appointments, medications, or even failed relationships!

ALTERNATIVES

As we continue to shine the spotlight on toxins around the home, try to look at this process in a positive light. There is a very good chance that something I'm about to mention here is stressing your system. Once we remove it, health automatically improves. Until we find that stressor, the smartest thing we can do is keep stacking the odds in your favor. We can do this by continuing to remove as many known toxic items from your environment as possible. Keep reading, because there is so much more to this book that just this chapter on toxins.

KITCHEN

A good place to find toxins in any home is in the kitchen. Look below your kitchen sink and you will find some of the deadliest of all household poisons. Many of these products contain carcinogenic ingredients. Carcinogenic simply means the substance or product has the potential to cause cancer. I'm stating the obvious here because I need you to make this connection when wiping down countertops. The last place we need carcinogenic chemicals is where we place our food!

I get it, we obviously need to clean our houses, but a less toxic option would be to use 3% hydrogen peroxide. You can buy this from any pharmacy. It's inexpensive and does a stellar job at killing bacteria, especially on countertops.

3%t hydrogen peroxide comes already diluted in the bottle. 3% percent hydrogen peroxide is quite a mild strength, it's NOT going to burn holes in your clothes, (that would be a different strength altogether). 3% is the same stuff that's sprayed on cuts and scrapes to clean them.

CUTTING BOARDS

For now, let's stick with household toxins found in the kitchen. Wooden cutting boards are said to trap 200x more bacteria than your toilet seat. (Ewh, now that's nasty.) When you spray 3% hydrogen peroxide on cutting boards, any bacteria will turn white and fizz. When you hear the fizz, it kinda lets you know hydrogen peroxide is doing its intended job. It also works pretty well if you get any meat/blood spills on the counter or in the fridge.

Use 3% hydrogen peroxide wherever you would a carcinogenic chemical. It's generally much safer around food than any of the usual household cleaners found in the store. You can even gargle with 3% hydrogen peroxide ... how many things under your sink would you do that with?

Remember that the skin is super absorbent. Anytime you hear the word "toxic" try to also hear the word "insidious". Those harsh toxic chemicals have the potential to build up over time.

TOILET

Rather than use a harsh toilet cleaner, alcohol can be just as effective at killing bacteria. Simply turn a regular bottle of (cheap) vodka into a spray by pouring it into a plastic spray bottle. Hey-presto, you now have an effective spray cleaner without any carcinogenic ingredients!

When it comes to cleaning glass, vinegar and newspaper cleans best, and without toxic side effects. You can use regular baking powder with a squirt of lemon to clean just about everything else!

AIR

Every time we let rip with that odor neutralizer we release a dangerous concoction of chemicals into the air. We like to think of air pollution as being an outdoor problem, but these types of sprays hang around in the air and irritate the lining of the lungs.

If you are looking to improve the overall air quality in your home/office/bedroom, then plants are an inexpensive way of doing it. NASA has detailed scientific research in this area bringing ample credibility to the topic.

Tip- If you don't have a green thumb, ask the sales assistant before you buy. Some plants are robust, others are picky. Getting this right in advance makes life just that little bit easier.

If your house smells for any reason, simply skip the harsh chemicals and open up a couple of windows, last time I checked, fresh air was still free!

Our lungs are important; we need them to work optimally as they form a vital part of the detoxification system. Continuing to breathe in harsh chemicals will irritate the delicate linings of the respiratory system.

COOKING

Be especially aware of any nonstick pans. Teflon or polytetrafluoroethylene (or PTFE for short) releases toxic gasses as it heats up. These toxic gasses have been linked to organ failure, reproductive damage, cancer and other harmful health effects. I know, right? Who makes this stuff?

Also, begin thinking about the oils you cook with. As a rule of thumb, if your frying pan is producing smoke while you cook, you are producing free radicals.

Free radicals are highly reactive uncharged molecules. Free radicals cause damage by adversely altering lipids, proteins, and even DNA. Prevention will always outperform cure, better to cook with avocado oil, clarified butter (ghee), or coconut oil. Generally speaking, these oils are better because they are more resistant to heating.

Oils to avoid at all costs are corn, canola, soybean, safflower and sunflower. These oils have unstable fats, which make an abundance of free radicals as well as destroying the nutritional properties of your food.

POTS & PANS

Aluminum saucepans were once quite popular. But we now know that trace amounts of aluminum can leach into the food as the pan heats up. When the amount of aluminum consumed exceeds the body's capacity to excrete it, illness follows. An added concern is that recent research has found high accumulations of aluminum in the brains of Alzheimer's patients. A good quality set of stainless steel pots and pans is a much better option.

LEAD

Lead is a known neurotoxin and dangerous heavy metal. Even in small amounts, lead can cause a wide range of serious health problems. As a side note, lead can also be found in many cosmetics. In recent years, government agencies have done a great job of alerting the public to the dangers of lead paint. The dangers of lead paint are real and far-reaching, and full credit where it's due — bravo to the environmental agency.

But if it's the goal of the government to steer us away from danger, why stop at lead? Why isn't the same level of attention being directed to other household toxic products such as the mercury found in light bulbs?

Many of these bulbs were pushed on to the unsuspecting public as a way to save energy. They are now declared so toxic that some local dumps won't take them. Check to see how many of those curly shaped light bulbs you have in your home. But be especially careful not to break one!

We have become so entwined with these toxic products that it's no longer possible to completely avoid them all. But we can minimize our personal exposure to them.

BATHROOM

Most people start their day by brushing their teeth, taking a shower and then rolling on some kind of underarm deodorant. Let's take a closer look at these daily occurrences.

When it comes to oral hygiene, it's hard to get away from fluoride. There's so much controversy already surrounding fluoride that I'm going to sidestep it all and leave you with this single thought ...

To function optimally your thyroid needs iodine. Iodine and fluoride appear on the same periodic table as halogens. This simply means that they are both chemically similar. Some believe that fluoride has the ability to block iodine absorption. That's a pretty big deal if you happen to be a thyroid.

Once the thyroid is compromised the whole body suffers. A daily hit of fluoride may have the potential to compound over time. Symptoms of a poorly functioning thyroid are fatigue, increased sensitivity to cold, heat, dry skin, and facial puffiness.

If enough of us make the switch, then perhaps corporations will begin to sit up and take notice. When it all seems too much, I like to think of it this way: we get to vote three times a day with the food we eat and maybe once a week with the toiletries we buy. Business follows the money, period.

Regular store bought shower gels and some soaps have toxic ingredients that can range from aluminum to parabens. In 2004, British cancer researcher Philippa Darbre Ph.D. found parabens present in malignant breast tumors. Parabens are well known to mimic/disrupt estrogen in the body and are found in many cosmetics.

Grab your shower gel, deodorant, makeup, and anything else that comes into contact with your skin. Look at the label of ingredients; a quick Google search should shock you to the core. Most well-stocked health food stores carry safer alternatives. We can all do our bit to stop these toxic invaders from seeping into our homes by switching to greener brands.

OFF-GASSING

Like any good detective, we are searching for clues in every corner of the house. It's worth noting that new furniture, rugs, and plastics ALL have the potential to "off-gas." Off-gassing (also known as outgassing) refers to the release of airborne particulates or chemicals. This is something to be aware of in a small bedroom, especially for those with young children.

Fire retardants can be particularly problematic. These can be found in your favorite armchair, on a mattress, and even in pillows. As pillows are next to our face for long periods, try to replace them with the least toxic option.

CARBON MONOXIDE

Let's not forget our old friend carbon monoxide which can come to our home through a faulty furnace. Carbon monoxide is sometimes referred to as the silent killer and yet detectors are incredibly easy to install. Compared to death (always a bummer), detectors offer good value for money.

RADON

The other sleeping giant to be on the lookout for is radon. Radon is a colorless, odorless, radioactive gas formed by the radioactive decay. Radon can lead to serious lung damage and is another known carcinogen.

Testing for radon is relatively easy and inexpensive. If a problem is detected, then installing a vent in the basement is usually the way to go. During the construction stage, a plastic membrane is sometimes added below the concrete.

EMFs

Okay, almost there. This is the last one before we start moving forward with a wide range of new and exciting topics.

EMF stands for Electromagnetic Field which is a field of energy created by electrically charged objects. The most common sources for high electromagnetic fields include proximity to power lines, transformers, and appliances. Sadly, it doesn't end there. Utility companies are now installing "smart" meters across the US which add to the frequency burden.

Wi-Fi and cellular phones release a fair share of dirty energy which has now become an omnipresent part of our lives. I fear the allure of technology is too great for me to overcome in one paragraph. Although I did once hear someone say, "If trees gave off a Wi-Fi signal we would all be out planting them; too bad they only produce the oxygen we breathe."

On the upside, for those of us who are surrounded by Wi-Fi routers from neighbors, it can be a perfect opportunity to say hi to them. Simply name your Wi-Fi network something like, "Mobile Police Surveillance" or "Shut Your Damned Dog Up."

My personal favorite is "Tell-my-Wi-Fi-Love-Her." Or if you are feeling particularly fresh, "Tell-**Your**-Wi-Fi love her". Lol.

What did we learn from this?

Toxins are an insidious part of everyday life that can take on many forms. We can influence the companies that make toxic products by buying from their green competitors.

Homework: Install a water filter and then replace all toxic cleaning substances with greener ones.

> Treat the earth well: it was *not* given to you by
> your parents, it was loaned to you by your children.
> – Ancient American Indian Proverb

Chapter 7

UNDERSTANDING SYMPTOMS

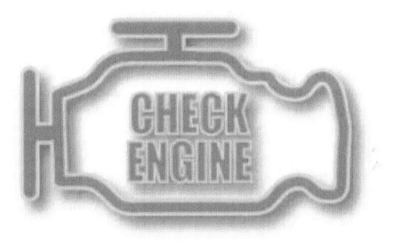

Symptoms let us know there is a problem in the body. The same way a vehicle Check Engine light might alert us to a problem under the hood. Symptoms offer us important clues that can guide us to solutions. Unfortunately, these clues are often silenced by prescription drugs such as painkillers.

If the prescription drug approach has worked for you in the past, then I suspect you wouldn't be reading this. For some, drugs do little to address the root cause of the problem. And so the underlying health problem rarely goes away.

LOOKING FOR CLUES

Back in the day, a good physician would carefully listen to a patient's concerns and then ask a series of probing questions. This is how good medicine was practiced and it helps uncover the root cause of a problem

Today, doctors are more inclined to use blood testing as a diagnostic tool. While this is not without merit, it's not infallible. Inevitably, some folks slip through the cracks. To add to the problem, the patient then leaves the doctor's office with an unresolved problem and a firm belief that they don't have a problem in that area. A good example of this is the thyroid TSH test, for reasons we will explore later.

If your symptoms remain unresolved there's a pretty good chance your doctor hasn't been listening to you. If this is you, grab a pencil and a blank sheet of paper.

For this exercise, we need to make a list of your current symptoms starting with the one that's the most problematic. Stay with me here, this is a simple but highly effective way of making sense of your medical maze.

Give this task some careful consideration as even minor things can later become important clues. If you aren't sure, just choose three health problems you wish you didn't have and write those down.

Don't get too freaked out if your list seems too short or too long. Everything in the body is connected. What ails you in one part of the body will logically throw up symptoms in another part. If you want to put this theory to the test, try dropping a hammer onto your big toe and see if your eyes water. Whoa, just kidding!

Okay, once your list is complete, check that all your symptoms are in order of priority, starting with whatever bothers you the most. Got it?

NOW BUILD A TIMELINE

Once you have that paper filled out, put it to one side and pull out a second blank sheet of paper. Only this time we are going to do something a little different. Turn the sheet of paper sideways (landscape orientation) and at the top write the word Timeline.

Now, look at your list of symptoms from the first sheet of paper.

The idea is to now transfer your symptoms onto the Timeline sheet in some kind of chronological order. It doesn't have to be perfect, at this stage we are just trying to get a sense of what went wrong and when.

Doing this on paper allows you to see patterns that you might otherwise have been missed. Yup, this a little effort on your part, but keep moving forward. The cost to you is low and the rewards can be high. It might just be the reason why no one else has figured out your annoying health problem.

Sometimes sleeping on it can help you fill any missing blanks. Asking your health care provider for a copy of your medical records can be helpful too. If you don't have access to your records, then don't panic. Progress is always better than perfection, just do the best you can with what information you have available.

Once you have your timeline sheet completed, take a while to look at it from different perspectives. Examine your it for patterns; maybe even ask a friend or relative to look over it with you.

UNTURNED STONES

Good police detectives leave no stones unturned. They often find evidence in the most unexpected places. If you want to be active in your own recovery treat it as if it were a crime scene. Your body is dying to give you these clues!

When filling out your timeline sheet, make a note of any recent medications, surgeries and/or medical procedures. Be aware that some of the side effects of medications can have lingering effects causing a disconnect in time.

Like any good detective, a simple process of elimination can be helpful. Pay particular attention to anything that's manmade or any unnatural occurrence in the body. When listing medications, don't forget to add things (if applicable) like the "humble" birth control pill. This alone has the potential to upset a woman's estrogen levels.

Try to keep an open mind when looking for patterns. Some people have been known to react to medications while others may even react to vitamins. Either way, both will have the same thing in common … a start date!

Be sure to add any recent dental visits to your timeline too. It's often said that health starts in the mouth but so too can illness. It's no secret that an abscessed tooth can be a drain on the entire immune system and the adrenal glands.

When looking for clues, don't be afraid to be guided by your intuition. Your intuition is probably the most underused tool you have at your disposal. Deep down you always know when something isn't right.

As we continue moving forward, let me again urge you to take your time and try not to feel overwhelmed. Your answer is in here somewhere.

FREAKY CLUES

Once you learn to look a little closer, you will notice clues are all around us. Here's an example of that.

I recently found myself in a hardware store and needed to speak to a sales assistant. He was a nice enough fellow and as I thanked him for his time I felt I should probably warn him about his high blood pressure. Left unchecked it can have deadly consequences.

He hadn't mentioned it during our short conversation so when I asked him how his high blood pressure was doing, he was actually quite surprised. He went on to say that he had only left the doctor's office that morning and had left with a diagnosis of hypertension (high blood pressure).

He knew he hadn't seen me at his doctor's office and by now he was curious to know how I had somehow picked up on it. Looking for clues had become such an ingrained habit of mine that I saw the answer right there in his fingernails. When a person has high blood pressure the half-moon shape at the base of the fingernails becomes quite prominent, (with the exception of the little finger which doesn't have a half moon at all). Surprised, he admitted he had never even noticed his fingernails before, and nor had his doctor.

Had he known what to look for earlier maybe he could have seen the warning signs coming? He was grateful that he now had a simple diagnostic tool (literally at his fingertips) for times when he couldn't get to his BP machine.

The fingernails alone can tell us about far more than just high blood pressure. Go ahead, take a look at the shape, color, and texture of your fingernails. Then check them against a friend's, you will quickly notice your fingernails are totally unique to you. Watch closely and you will see that your fingernails also change over time, and they *always* tell a story.

TIMING

Timing is everything in this life, we have to be aware that some people want to hear these insights, and some people don't. My wife recently met with some of her knitting friends and dragged me along for the ride. During introductions, I shook hands with a middle-aged lady and immediately noticed she had dry skin. I also noted that she was the only person wearing a sweater in a room full of people wearing T-shirts. A quick glance at her eyebrows revealed that the outer third of her eyebrow had completely thinned out too. Hmm, I see.

As I watched her crunch on her second cup of ice within fifteen minutes, I wondered if the root of this lady's obvious thyroid problem was anemia. People sometimes crave ice when they are low in iron.

As I sat quietly observing from across the room my wife came over and discreetly reminded me of the agreement we had made earlier. It went something like this … "These are my knitting friends, try not to freak any of them out." My point? Clues are all around us, and they are helpful, but sometimes so too is an element of discretion. Lol.

What did we learn from this?
Symptoms are important clues that should be investigated rather than suppressed. If you are stuck on that merry-go-round of illness it's absolutely okay to play a bigger role in your own recovery. Nobody knows your situation better than you do.

Homework: Create your own Timeline of symptoms and look at it objectively.

Chapter 7a

BONUS CHAPTER

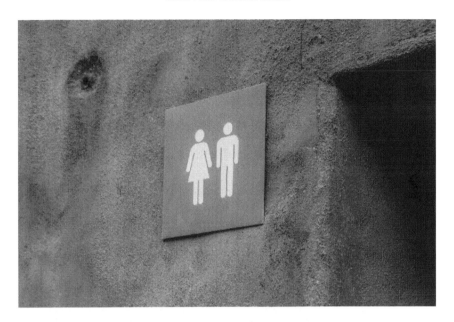

If we eat a balanced diet, we can expect to expel a stool every day. The size, shape, color, and texture of the stool all tell an interesting story.

If you felt this got a little too weird too quick, then you might want to hold onto your hat because more is coming. I've also saved the best (or weirdest) for last).

Diet, certain medications, and even vitamins can all change the color of stool. A "normal" stool should be somewhere on the brown spectrum. This is a sure sign that the liver is excreting enough bile. Think of bile as dishwasher detergent helping to clean excess grease from the dishes. In its most basic form, bile is doing the very same thing. It's helping your stomach deal with all that grease, fat and oil found in certain foods.

It should come as no surprise that nutrition is inextricably tied to digestive health and many of these issues are diet related. Good digestion always starts in the mouth. To help you remember this, think of it this way: the better you chew, the better the poo. That said, if you are experiencing any form of discomfort or pain then it's important to get yourself checked out by a healthcare professional.

They say a picture is worth a thousand words. With that in mind, the Bristol Stool Chart below shows better in pictures what I am attempting to describe in words.

BRISTOL STOOL CHART

	Type 1	Separate hard lumps	**SEVERE CONSTIPATION**
	Type 2	Lumpy and sausage like	**MILD CONSTIPATION**
	Type 3	A sausage shape with cracks in the surface	**NORMAL**
	Type 4	Like a smooth, soft sausage or snake	**NORMAL**
	Type 5	Soft blobs with clear-cut edges	**LACKING FIBRE**
	Type 6	Mushy consistency with ragged edges	**MILD DIARRHEA**
	Type 7	Liquid consistency with no solid pieces	**SEVERE DIARRHEA**

Constipation can be a sign of an underperforming thyroid. If you are on the thyroid merry-go-round check out my link at the bottom of this post. It's actually not uncommon for the TSH test to give a false reading.

A normal stool shouldn't stink up the bathroom, and if it has you hanging your head out the bathroom window then it could be a sign of malabsorption. A stool with lots of holes drilled into it could be a sign of a parasitic infection which can rob your body of vital nutrients. Here's where it gets interesting.

PEE

The color of your urine offers invaluable clues to what's happening inside. Healthy-looking pee should be the color of straw. If the color is clear, then it's passing through your kidneys a little too quickly. If this happens on a regular basis, then it may be prudent to get it checked out.

If your pee is dark, it could be a sign you are dehydrated. If it's dark orange and you are passing pale stools it could be a sign of a malfunctioning liver. If this is you, pay close attention to the whites of your eyes which may also begin to show a yellow tint. The liver and kidneys are organs to help us rid the body of toxins and it's important to have them working optimally.

If pee is cloudy or murky it could be a sign of kidney stones forming. As a rule, you won't have to second guess when stones are ready to expel as the pain to the kidney will be excruciating. Kidney stones can sometimes be related to problems with the parathyroid. Although the parathyroid and thyroid are both located in the same area of the body, they perform very different jobs. The primary job of the parathyroid is to regulate the body's calcium levels.

Again, medications, vitamins, and diet can change the color, but in most cases, if pee is cloudy, murky, and foul smelling it could be a sign that you have a UTI (urinary tract infection). If diabetes is suspected the kidneys will do their best to get rid of excess glucose and the pee may smell sweet. If you really want to put this to the test, you could try tasting the urine rather than doing the finger prick test. Whoa! Hang on, I didn't say you had to drink it, I said taste it.

Before people start jumping all over me on this, might I point out that whenever survival expert Bear Grylls drinks his own pee on national T.V he quickly becomes the darling of the day. Diabetes is a serious illness that can lead to all sorts of complications. If this simple technique brings attention to this issue, then it lets not be in a rush to dismiss it.

I know to some this may all seem a little gross, but the aim here isn't to tickle your ears with things that are pleasant to hear, it's to help you stay well. Once you get over the mental hang-up of checking your pee and poop for clues, it can be a highly effective diagnostic tool. Remember, nobody knows your situation better than you do and it's okay to play a bigger role in your own recovery.

What did we learn from this?
Pee and poop offer us important clues to our internal health.

Chapter 8

DEBUNKING THE BAD GENES THEORY

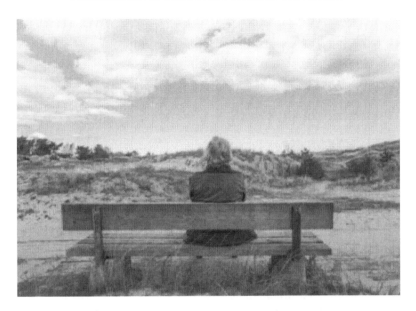

Recently, I visited my elderly aunt in a nursing home. It soon became clear that she had no clue who I was, or even where she was. This once dignified woman was now trapped inside a sickly body. Her days spent relying on others to prevent her from sitting in cold, damp underwear.

As I looked around the nursing home I quickly noticed that my aunt's situation was being replicated. Withered bodies sitting in front of mind-numbing television sets feeding on spoonful of mush. Seeing people like this weighed heavy on my soul.

On the opposite end of this spectrum meet 102-year-old Edie Simms of Missouri. Edie should be an inspiration to us all. In her long life she's had many experiences, but getting arrested was not one of them.

For her 102nd birthday, Edie decided to turn herself into the local police department — evidently, it was on her bucket list. As she walked to the waiting squad car, Edie also requested that she be handcuffed.

After more than a hundred years, Edie's mind remains as sharp as a tack. Prior to her arrest, Edie had spent much of her time offering support to the "younger" residents at the senior home. Helping others has been Edie's formula for living a long and productive life.

Unfortunately, minds like Edie's are now becoming few and far between. While there are lots of theories for this, it's important to recognize that our brains are hard-wired to be of service to others.

Science is now able to demonstrate how a part of the brain known as the subgenual anterior cingulate cortex, lights up whenever we help others. Although after 102 years, I suspect Edie already knew this. On the flip side of Edie's story sits senile dementia.

Alzheimer's Disease International estimates that the number of people living with dementia will double every 20 years. That's 74.7 million lives devastated by 2030 and whopping 131 million by 2050.

Health problems aren't confined to the older generation. Some estimates suggest that a child born in the U.S. today will have a lower life expectancy than those in the generation before.

BAD GENES

The presumption by some is that our ancestors must have somehow given us bad genes. Personally, I take issue with this argument more than any other.

Why?

First, when a patient is told they have "bad genes" it suggests that they are powerless to control their own destiny. This type of thinking instills a negative mindset which is not only unhelpful, it's also deeply flawed.

Second, the human body is a highly complex marvel with the ability to repair itself. The way we perceive this remarkable phenomenon is essential for longevity and recovery.

The belief that we are predisposed to illness through our ancestors' genes doesn't take into account the toxic world we have made for ourselves. Today, most of the water we drink comes to us from a plastic bottle. And the food we eat is highly processed and often loaded with toxic additives and excess sugars.

Spend enough time sitting in your doctor's office, and you may hear that your suffering is genetic. In case you missed it, this little gem hints that you are somehow to blame for your illness. This way of thinking presents a much bigger problem for you than it does to the doctor treating you.

Let's look at it this way. If your mom ate junk food for breakfast, lunch, and dinner then as a kid so did you. When both become diabetic does anyone stop to ask if this predisposition a result of bad genes or simply a bad diet?

The short answer to that question is probably going to be no, in part because doctors receive so little training in the field of nutrition. Now we start to see a very different picture and one that challenges the concept that our cause is lost to bad genes.

The "bad" genes hypothesis glosses over a vast array of toxic environmental factors. If you grew up in cramped squalor and suffered from head lice, then so did your siblings. If you grew up in a home full of mold, there is a pretty good chance you developed chest problems and so did your siblings. If you grew up in a house next to a toxic waste dump, then so did your siblings. When elevated rates of cancer show up in these tight family units, does anyone ever stop to ask why?

When we apply a little lateral thinking, the problem begins to look a lot less like genetics and more like common sense. Let's not forget that our ancestors' genes must have been pretty robust to survive. Perhaps those medical pundits are referring to our ancestors from a hundred years ago? Let's take a look.

WORLD WAR ONE

We owe our freedom to those souls who bravely gave up their lives to the First World War. It's well documented that during that time more good men lost their lives to poor sanitation than to enemy machine gun fire!

Wait a second … are you catching this?

I'm saying that between 1914 and 1918 a plumber's wrench could have saved more lives the surgeon's scalpel!

Today we know that the spread of harmful bacteria can be slowed down with effective hand washing. Hence we have all become overly obsessed with doing it. If only more men had been given access to hot water and soap, fewer deaths would have resulted.

NO SHIT

Before we allow science to poke a finger at our ancestors' genes, let us remind ourselves that poor waste management and disease go hand in hand.

When we look at communicable diseases, it's worth noting that indoor toilets were once considered a luxury. Right up to the late nineteenth century, "soil-men" were being employed to remove human waste from our homes and businesses.

Typically, this was done at night and by hand by a four-man team consisting of a hole man, a rope man, and two tubmen. The hole man crawled into the cesspool and filled the buckets. The rope man hauled up the buckets full of human waste and passed them to the two tubmen who put them on the truck. These poor unfortunate souls carried these buckets of slopping waste all night long — now that's what you call a shitty job.

As for the spills? They were often left in the yard where young children played during the day.

In pre-sewer America, open sewage carts were being pushed along with human excrement dripping over the sides. On a hot summer's day, it's often said that the stench would hang in the air making people gag as they scurried away.

When we look back at disease, let's not be in a rush to discount the obvious advantages of the modern flushing toilet. Polio is often spread via the stool of an infected person. If we put our reality goggles on, it could be argued that plumbers are again saving lives. As sanitation continued to improve your ancestors' genes not only went on to survive, they positively thrived. Hoorah, for indoor plumbing and hot showers!

So where does this all fit in?

Today we face a new threat from pesticides, pollution, parabens, plastics, and other petroleum-based products (and that's just the letter P). To blame our toxic world on our ancestors' genes is not only incorrect, it's actually a little insulting to them.

No?

Okay, let's try this.

Regardless of your ethnicity, your DNA stretches countless generations. Perhaps even back to the Roman empire.

From the intense heat of North Africa to the cold and damp of Northern England, Roman soldiers marched around in full body armor. After weeks of marching, these formidable warriors then had to contend with a ferocious fight to the death. No, last bus home, no cough drops from the pharmacy.

If our ancestors' genes were so predisposed to weakness, how did they manage to survive any of this?

Imagine if right now, you and I found ourselves on a battlefield standing toe-to-toe with a fully kitted-out Roman soldier. As we struggle to lift the 65 pounds of body armor, how do you think we would fair?

I think we are about to get our toxic butts kicked by our ancestors.

THOSE STUFFY VICTORIANS

Maybe the blame for all of our problems lies with those stuffy, oh-so-proper Victorians. But compare those trim Victorian body shapes to our high obesity rates of today, perhaps once again, our ancestors got a lot of things right.

But it's not only the physical. Our modern-day stressed out ADD brains struggle to compare to those of our Victorian ancestors. It's easy to see how their minds worked from the things that they built. To this day, Victorian architecture is a testament to the meticulous craftsmen involved in building them.

Today, we are quick to build soul-less metal boxes. Although metal boxes are a good fit for industrial units, they have a distinct emphasis on cheapness rather than quality.

Which begs the question. How far has our current standard fallen, if the generation we once considered to be the "unwashed masses" is still outperforming us today?

Rest assured, whatever is going is wrong here hasn't got a whole lot to do with your great-grandparents. Seems to me our ancestors handed us some pretty good genes.

Maybe if we embraced our ancestral genes rather than blame them for our modern diseases we could begin to create a better world for ourselves.

What did we learn from this?
Squalid living conditions and a lack of personal hygiene have always
played a pivotal role in disease. These are well-documented historical
facts.

Clearly, our ancestors got a lot of things right and maybe we shouldn't be
in a rush to leave them buried in the past. To accomplish what they did,
our early ancestors must have been a pretty hearty bunch. By
comparison, we now seem hell-bent on making ourselves extinct.

So let us now look for solutions.

Chapter 9

THE CORNERSTONE OF GOOD HEALTH

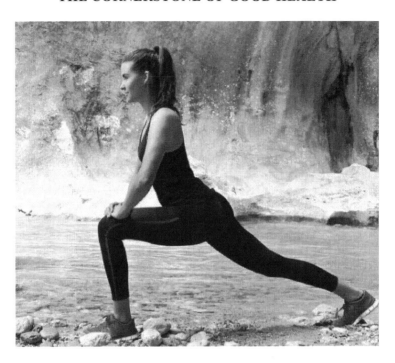

The human body has eleven systems, one of them is quite remarkable in the fact that you get to choose how well it works. Before we explore this system in more detail, let's take a quick look at the other ten.

We have a skeletal system, muscular system, respiratory system, immune system, reproductive system, endocrine system, circulatory system, nervous system, excretory system and the integumentary system. If you aren't sure what that last one looks like, take a look in the mirror; it's everything you see on the outside of your skin, nails, hair, etc.

That's ten, any idea which system is missing?

This last final system has the potential to make or break your health. More illness begins here than anywhere else in the body. But you can choose to enhance this system or continue to damage it. That's good news for anyone looking to have greater influence over their health because this system is the very cornerstone of good health.

Without further ado, it's the digestive system! — Perhaps we should have gone with a drum roll.

Why?

Think about it, the digestive system is home to a whopping 75+% of our immune system. If that hasn't just knocked you off your seat, let's try saying it another way…. Death begins in the colon. *I know, right? Bummer.*

But the fun doesn't stop there. Gut bacteria manufacture the majority of the brain's supply of serotonin. Wait a second, are you catching this?

Serotonin is a chemical that's responsible for maintaining positive mood balance. Perhaps this is why the digestive system is often referred to as the body's second brain.

The digestive system is heavily affecting all other systems and yet we think of depression and anxiety as something that affects only the mind. *Hmm, I see.*

AND THE NOT SO GOOD NEWS

Statistically speaking, many health problems have their roots planted in the gut. To be clear, these problems aren't confined to bloating or gas. Hell no, those are just basic clues to tell us we are doing something wrong, the overall issue is much bigger. These are by no means limited to hormonal problems, diabetes, chronic fatigue, inflammation, fibromyalgia, eczema, rosacea, anxiety, depression, Crohn's disease, IBS, and celiac disease. Some evidence even suggests that autoimmune diseases such as Hashimoto's and rheumatoid arthritis play out in the gut.

I know what you are thinking because I thought. If the gastrointestinal tract (GI tract for short) is behind so much potential illness why is it going wrong?

The job of the GI tract isn't to cause illness, make no mistake, the GI tract is not some dumbass design that suddenly decided to malfunction. It's alive and intelligent; perhaps this is why we often have "gut-feelings" about certain things. To save any confusion, let's define what the GI tract is.

In its most basic form, the job of the GI tract is to digests foods, absorbing nutrients, and expel waste. That's its job. It starts at point A (the mouth) and ends at point B (the anus). What happens between depends on the choices you make. This is your job.

DO THIS

Humor me, for the next 24 hours write down EVERYTHING you swallow, be it solid, fluid, vitamin, or pharmaceutical drug. If you need to, carry a small pocket-sized notebook around so you don't miss anything. The next morning take a hard look at what you wrote. Something on that list is a problem; I just know it is. The aim of this next section is to help you find out what.

Your digestive system is smart but it's not magical. If you put garbage in, garbage comes out. The digestive system can only work with the raw materials you give it. Everything we put into the digestive system is a choice, nobody forces us to buy heavily processed foods. Food is the fuel your body runs on — whether its carrots, cucumbers, or chips. This, in turn, is then fed to your cells.

Indian medicine and Chinese medicine date back thousands of years. Both regard the digestive system to be the cornerstone of all health. By comparison, western medicine offers little in the form of nutritional training to its junior doctors. Given the explosion in both Type 2 diabetes and obesity, we might expect new doctors to be given more nutritional training, not less.

Wait a second, are you catching this?

Science-based medicine doesn't value nutrition enough to train its doctors extensively in this field. I know right, WTF? (Where's-The-Food)

HOSPITAL FOOD

This lack of nutritional training creates an obvious disservice to the patients they aim to treat. To take this a step further, we could argue that hospitals should be the one place where food is the absolute best money can buy. Sadly, it does little to nourish a body trying to recover from illness.

To be fair to the medical profession, I've yet to meet a doctor without a bright mind. These dedicated men and women are gifted in so many ways and yet results are often stifled by adopting a flawed approach to nutrition. Let's not forget, this isn't a new concept, 430 years B.C. Hippocrates was wandering around and saying outrageous things like:

ALL disease begins in the gut –Hippocrates

Personally, I believe most doctors are smart enough to figure this out for themselves. But for them to veer away from a path they were trained to follow can attract criticism from their peers.
During my own brush with serious illness, I was sometimes hooked up to some pretty fancy machines costing thousands of dollars. Yet the whole time no one ever thought to look me in the eye to say, "Hey, quick question for you sir, what type of fuel are you running your body on?" For all they knew, I could have been stuffing my face twelve times a day with Twinkies… just sayin'. I *wasn't* but the point I'm making is this- the importance of diet wasn't on anyone's radar.

THE BIG SQUEEZE

These days we ride our digestive systems pretty hard and to be fair it's doing exactly what we ask of it. It doesn't matter what we swallow, everything is pulled apart and squeezed in an attempt to extract nutrients.

These nutrients then run along the sides of the intestine wall where millions of tiny finger-like projections called villi are waiting to absorb them. Once all key nutrients have been extracted, any leftovers get sent out as waste (AKA poop).

Keep in mind that villi are extremely sensitive. This is good news if you have just eaten a bowl of homemade kale soup, and not so great if you have just eaten chocolate flavored bacon chips washed down with a diet coke. Despite there being lots of misinformation out there, I'm sure many already knew this.

Astonishingly enough, the standard food pyramid is heavily influenced by the corporations who stand to benefit from the foods they recommend. Low fat, and high sugar spring to mind.

To recap, the whole GI tract is an incredibly delicate organ. If we feed it foods it likes, life is good. If we feed it foods that are laced with antibiotics, harmful additives, excessive sugars, pesticides, and growth hormones our reward is health problems.

I mentioned that the digestive system is the cornerstone of all health, right?

There is an unmistakable correlation between how we treat the GI tract and how it reacts. Treat it well and it will serve you well. This isn't rocket science, you can't put bad things into it and expect good things to come out.

Almost two and a half thousand years later, Hippocrates is back again. He said it this way: "The bodily process of digestion and absorption is one of the most important to our health." Today this statement appears truer than ever.

Symptoms present themselves as the body's way of trying to get our attention. Constipation, bloating, acid reflux, gas, and stomach pain are all signs that the GI tract is no longer tolerating our poor food choices. I hate to be the one to tell you, but your gut doesn't like all those GMO grains you keep forcing it to deal with. I know right, WTF? (Who's-The-Farmer?)

Grains are found in things like bread, cereal, and pasta but they also sneak into lots of other products. Grains are the seed of the crop, and nature designed these seeds to survive if something came along and ate them.

Maybe that is the reason gluten can be so problematic for certain people. Hello gluten types. Although, this can be a much wider issue than just gluten, here's why.

GLUTEN-FREE? — Meh

Often when people go gluten-free they exchange one grain for a different one. Unfortunately, that doesn't work out too well. Grain, is still grain, switching out wheat bread for rice bread is no different than quitting one brand of cigarettes and exchanging it for another. So let's flush this one out while I still have your attention. It's not just gluten that's causing the problem, ALL grains can be harsh on the digestive system.

CORN

Grains also have a twisted cousin and it goes by the name of corn. Corn is similar to grain in that it was designed by nature to be a part of the plant's reproductive system. It's a seed, for that reason, corn is notoriously difficult to digest. Corn is cheap to produce and is often used in food as a filler. Adding to the problem, 90% of all corn is now genetically modified. But even organic corn can be harsh on the digestive system, often times it will pass through the digestive system intact. Obviously eliminating these products from your diet today would be a step in the right direction.

Think of food as fuel for the body and then take responsibility for the way you eat rather than handing the responsibility over to the supermarket.

Rather than letting this overwhelm you, let's look at this as a positive. You have now identified two of the biggest players for causing digestive issues. Grains and corn. What you choose to do with this information is now up to you.

What did we learn from this?
The digestive system deserves a little respect; it plays a huge role in making or breaking your health. Numerous health problems begin first in the gut.

Homework: make a comprehensive list of anything that passes your lips over the next 24 hours.

Chapter 10

IT TAKES GUTS TO LEAK

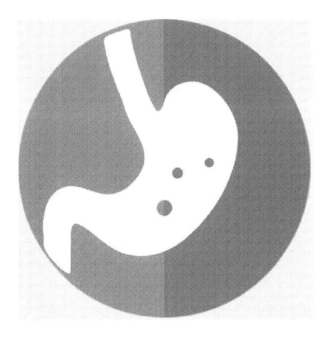

In your mind's eye, imagine holding a bicycle inner tube. Next, take a pair of scissors and cut the tube so that it hangs down in a single straight line. Then place the tube on the floor in front of you. What you now have is a design very similar to your digestive system. Both are hollow tubes with an opening at the top (the mouth) and an exit at the bottom (anus).

If we forced food into the top of the inner tube and then squeezed it all the way down, it would eventually come out at the bottom. This would be a pretty good example of how the body expels waste. Now hold that image.

Again take out our scissors and begin making several microscopic nicks to the inner-tube. If we again try to force the food down the tube notice how some of it begins to squeeze through those tiny nicks. In theory, those tiny particles are now finding their way into the bloodstream. That's not good, right?

Not really. The immune system is smart but it isn't expecting to see fecal matter and particles of food floating around in the bloodstream. As far as the immune system is concerned, all partially digested bacon sandwiches are safely trapped inside the inner tube (AKA your digestive tract).

So when the immune system spots something it doesn't recognize, it gets a little freaked out and sends the whole system into red alert. Boomshakalaka, say hello to your new food sensitivities.

But guts aren't meant to leak so why would they do that?

In certain individuals, proteins found in gluten can be notoriously difficult to break down. Over time, the delicate lining of the gut can become irritated and inflamed. Once the lining becomes permeable food particles to ooze through and enter the bloodstream (as with our inner-tube example). The term for this is often described as leaky gut syndrome. Let's explore this concept.

From the time we swallow it, to the time it leaves the body, food was always meant to stay inside the digestive system. For it to wander into the bloodstream is both unusual and unnatural. Some might say, almost as unnatural as the way we now grow our food.

In recent years, food has recently undergone some pretty radical changes. Much of our food is now sprayed with some pretty heavy-duty pesticides. This has become an everyday farming practice and nobody seems to mind. Yet, many of these pesticides contain EDCs (endocrine disrupting chemicals). They work by disrupting the central nervous systems of bugs. Some of the newer insecticides also work by disrupting the guts of insects. Hmm, I see.

The standard western diet is also heavily reliant on grain, most of which have now been "modified" to increase crop yields. While this may sound good, nobody can say for sure how this will affect the human race long term.

For some of us, the gluten found in wheat, barley, and rye is already causing a wide range of reactions. These reactions can range from a feeling of general fatigue to mental confusion and just about everything in between. Throw into the mix a few thousand food additives and we shouldn't be all that surprised when people experience digestive issues.

Once grains become a problem, switching to "gluten-free" products are unlikely to solve the problem. Think of a lung cancer patient switching different cigarette brands as a way of limiting symptoms. Once your immune system reacts to gluten, you may need to go grain free or you may find you are simply exchanging one problem for another.

The good news is you can buy certified gluten-free oats, but it pays to be sure of the source. The bad news is some people are still going to react because cross-contamination with gluten is common during processing.

INFLAMMATION

It's important to note that inflammation plays a pivotal role in ALL illness. When your immune system begins to attack food particles in the bloodstream, systemic inflammation is your reward.

A small amount of localized inflammation can be thought of as a well-guarded campfire with a practical benefit. But, inflammation left to linger can soon become a rampant forest fire. The connection between illness and this type of out of control inflammation is well documented.

It seems that doctors are better equipped to hand out pills than they are dietary advice. But they do agree that gluten has the potential to cause damage to the intestinal lining. When the intestines become inflamed it can be harder for the body to absorb nutrients.

Many of us have been conditioned to think the answer to our health problems lies in swallowing more pills. But trying to medicate our way out of a poor diet is just poor judgment.

Keep in mind that the pharmaceutical industry is like no other. It generates higher profit margins than the oil industry. Big pharma has no interest in your nutritional needs. So the mere mention of a leaky gut in your physician's office and you can expect an uncomfortably long stare.

If you have been paying close attention you may have noticed that the keyword I keep using to describe these events is "theory." You might now be asking why this is still a theory? Well, clinical trials cost millions of dollars and this "theory" simply isn't sexy enough to pay for those clinical trials. Put simply, there's no money to be made from telling you to change your diet.

With so many diseases currently labeled "unknown," perhaps the leaky gut theory should be given a little more merit. Or, at the very least, explored to the fullest. Some of the best ideas start out as just that, a theory.

Here's a remarkable story of doctor Ignaz Semmelweis. It begins in 1846 when he took his first medical position as an appointed assistant in a maternity ward at Vienna General Hospital. Shortly after doing so he noticed that some wards had a disproportionately higher infant mortality rate than others.

Ward one gained a particularly bad reputation and many local women preferred to give birth in the street. Statistically speaking, their chances of survival actually improved. Young doctor Semmelweis was told by his seniors that the reason for these higher deaths in ward 1 was a "poisonous gas" that often came into the ward. But doctor Semmelweis had his own theory and was quick to notice something quite odd.

Ward one (the maternity ward) was directly next to the mortuary! It was a common practice for doctors to perform autopsies in the morning and then work in Ward number one in the afternoon.

Back then, hygiene wasn't properly understood and a scalpel used in an autopsy was often later used to cut an umbilical cord. Even basic hand washing wasn't in place until Dr. Semmelweis introduced it as a standard protocol.

But here's the rub.

Despite an immediate reduction in deaths, the views held by Dr. Semmelweis were not part of the general medical beliefs. He was not attacked by senior medical figures and later dismissed from his position. I know, right? But keep reading, it gets even worse.

With Dr. Semmelweis out of the way, ward number one soon went back to its old ways. Not surprisingly fatality rates immediately returned to their level pre-1847. It takes courage to challenge such embedded belief but Dr. Semmelweis was enraged by such ignorance. He even wrote open letters to his main critics calling them "ignorant murderers."

LEST WE FORGET

And so, for the next 20 years, Dr. Semmelweis did everything he could to warn people. But people refused to believe that dead bodies had germs. Doctors continued to deliver babies without washing their hands.

Unfortunately, the status quo had just about enough of doctor Dr. Semmelweis his germ theory. In 1865 he was tricked into visiting a mental asylum. When he tried to leave, Dr. Semmelweis was forcibly restrained and put in a straitjacket. His injuries were such that they became infected and two weeks later he died. Dr. Semmelweis was buried in Vienna and very few people attended his funeral. Today his theory is still saving lives. Perhaps in time we will look back and find that the leaky gut "theory" also had merit.

Those who do not learn history are doomed to repeat it – George Santayana

I appreciate that some readers may have quite a comprehensive understanding of these concepts already. While others may be hearing these things for the very first time. In either case, my goal is to present information in a way that's easy to absorb.

IT'S NOT YOUR FAULT

You might not hear this all that often, but the poor food choices you make are not entirely your fault. You should be able to go to the supermarket and pick out anything on the shelf to nourish the body. But somewhere along the line, everything got twisted. Supermarket foods are now high in calories but low in nutritional content. They also contain a fair share of colorings, preservatives, artificial flavors, high fructose corn syrup and food additives. As a rule of thumb, if you can't pronounce the words on the label, then your intestines aren't going to like it.

This begs the question, what's up with food?

Recently I was once at my local food store and noticed an elderly lady in the parking lot struggling to load a heavy grocery bag into her car. It took me but a second to help lift the bag into her trunk and she was duly thankful. As she drove away waving, it made me wonder if she fully understood the meaning of words like acesulfame-K, Aspartame, and monosodium glutamate.

With so many toxic food additives, it can be a full-time job trying to keep up with them. Perhaps the onus shouldn't be on the shopper to have to read the fine print on every label.

The hard way is to read every label; the easy way is not to buy food with labels. I know right, it's a radical concept. Better hold onto your hat, more is coming.

You may view your local supermarket as a convenience, but remember it's a business, and as such, it is there to make money. If the supermarket is creating meaningful jobs and making it easy for you to gather food, that's great. But someone needs to ask, why can't we just go back to having simple ingredients that are less harmful to our body?

While we wait for the supermarkets to do the right thing, the good news is that if you get to vote with your feet three times a day. The bad news is it's actually easier to buy crack cocaine on the street than it is to buy locally raised organic chicken. What's up with that?

If you aren't sure what to buy or where to buy it, no need to panic — I'm here to help. Just keep reading my posts and all will become clear.

BE KIND TO YOUR SMALL INTESTINE

For this next exercise, you will need a small cloth tape measure like the one found in a sewing kit. Got one? … Great.

Today more than ever we spend a disproportionate amount of our time sitting down; we do it in our cars, at our desks, at the movies, even while we eat. Hell, you are probably doing it right now!

While sitting down, grab that cloth tape measure and run it around your waist and make a note of the number. Now stand up and do the same thing. What you should have is two very different numbers, am I right?

Now take off your pants (trousers to my European homies) and measure the inside of the waistband. Forget what the label says, just measure it and then write that number down. Finally, do the same thing with your underwear while in the "unstretched" position.

Now compare all four sets of numbers. Do you see it? Your clothes are restricting the free movement of your small intestine for sixteen hours a day. Throw in a few leather belts and buckles and we really compound the problem. If you suffer from bloating this whole restrictive process will be magnified tenfold, especially when you are sitting.

The goal here is to try to avoid unnecessary discomfort to the small intestine. Keep in mind that the accurate sizing of our clothes depends largely on who made them. It can be a costly mistake to simply grab "your" size and go. Always take the time to try new clothes on in a sitting position. Also, be aware that our body shapes can change from season to season, it's not uncommon to gain a few pounds in the winter.

Your digestive system needs you to wear clothes that are comfortable. If you happen to be wearing ultra-skinny jeans, then this news is no doubt falling on deaf ears. Organ compression can lead to serious digestive problems down the road. I'd really like to prevent that from happening to you. Try to keep in mind that hospital gowns can be less flattering than jeans.

Now go burn those skinny jeans.

What did we learn from this?
Many of the great medical discoveries were first mocked by the medical establishment.

For the sake of your digestive system, consider buying whole foods that come without any labels to read.

Homework: Check out Dr. Darren Schmidt's short video on leaky gut. His videos are always a breath of fresh air. Here's the link, enjoy! https://www.youtube.com/watch?v=j1T5LLfk6L8

Chapter 11

ALKALIZE TO ENERGIZE

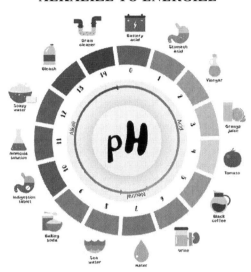

While we are all uniquely different, we all share one thing in common — our blood needs to be slightly alkaline to stay healthy. But what does that mean and how do we do it?

For anyone looking to enjoy better health, the following information is important to know. The difference between life and death often hangs on the body's ability to manage our pH levels.

To help us measure the states of acidic to alkaline we use numbers ranging from zero to fourteen. The lower the number, the more acidic, the higher the number, the more alkaline. For example, battery acid would be around 0 and household ammonia around 12. The number 7 is represented as neutral — neither acidic nor alkaline. But the margin for error in the human body is remarkably small.

The body strives to keep our blood pH around 7.35 to 7.45 (slightly alkaline). Generally, the body does an excellent job of keeping things tightly regulated. But even the slightest difference can dramatically impact our health.

Once blood has excessive acidity it goes by the name of acidosis. Acidosis can quickly lead to serious health conditions and even death. The American Association for Clinical Chemistry (AACC) categorizes acidosis as lower than 7.35. If you stop and think about it, that's really not that far away from 7.45.

Obviously, we don't want to be too acidic, nor do we want to be too alkaline. Here's why.

When the pH of the blood becomes too alkaline it is referred to as alkalosis. Alkalosis occurs above 7.45, again bringing with it a whole host of health problems. We aren't even two minutes into this post and already we know that blood pH has a narrow range of 7.35 to 7.45 and stepping outside of those parameters brings BIG trouble. Try to remember these sets of numbers, before this story ends I'll ask you about them. It's actually quite common for most people to get the answer wrong.

So by now, you are probably thinking, if this whole pH thing is so important, what the heck keeps it in balance? That's a really great question and I like the way you are starting to think. It's sometimes said that knowledge is having all the right answers, but intelligence is asking the right questions.

The pH of the body is kept within this range in part by the kidneys and lungs. When the body becomes too acidic, the kidneys help restore balance by using common electrolytes — sodium, potassium, magnesium, calcium, plus chloride, phosphates, and sulfates, yadda, yadda, yadda — to buffer acidity. This buffering system is what keeps you alive.

Here's the rub. If the body remains in an acidic state for any length of time, minerals used to buffer that acidity becomes depleted. The body doesn't want you to die from an excess of acidity. It will do whatever it takes to stop the blood pH from slipping below 7.35.

Can you see the problem yet?

When the body runs short of available minerals, it's forced to take drastic action. It does this by stealing minerals from the bones, cells, organs, and tissues. This isn't an ideal situation and should be thought of as the body pulling the emergency brake to keep you alive.

Minerals are critical to our health. Not only to buffer acidity but also to keep the cells functioning optimally. Cells devoid of minerals cannot dispose of waste or oxygenate. From head to toe, our bodies are made up of cells. Do you see the importance of this yet?

A lack of minerals will hinder the absorption of vitamins and allow toxins and pathogens to accumulate in the body. Ultimately this will lead to a suppressed immune system. All of this stems from a body striving to keep itself from becoming too acidic. I know what you are thinking because I've had the same thought. What would make the body too acidic, am I right?

STRESS

There are several factors and one of these is stress. But as we all know too well, stress is an omnipresent part of life that we can't always get away from. The best we can do is manage it. At times, that's easier said than done.

We all get stressed but the good news is we can adopt strategies for reducing stress. If you find yourself doing a job you hate to surround yourself with more things, then it might be worth re-evaluating what's really important to you. More stuff, or more health? When stress gets to the point where it's making you ill, then you have the right to choose another path. Sometimes owning less stuff can lead to more health.

DEAD

I once made this same point to an elderly Scotsman who happened to be a retired accountant. As I watched him work himself into the ground I joked with him there are no pockets in a shroud. I did my best to assure him that he couldn't take any of his money with him. He looked me squarely in the eye and said, "Son, if I can't take it with me then I'm not going." Either way, he's dead now so I guess I was right and he was wrong.

As in this case, stress can be self-inflicted, but it can also come from the people with whom we surround ourselves. Maybe you have a toxic friend in your life that's adding to your stress — some people are just wired that way. You can't change them, but you can change your exposure to them. And I suspect deep down you already know this.

Given the importance of this topic, you may find it helpful to periodically check your pH. This is inexpensive to do and you can easily do this from home. For this test you will need to buy a set of pH testing strips, often sold in your local health food store. The kit comes with litmus paper that you will pee on. Simply match the sample test strip with the various color shades found on the box.

There is a right way to do this and a wrong way.

The wrong way is to pee on them as soon as you get them home. Rushing to do the test will always give you a false reading, so it's a waste of both the litmus strips and your time.

The right way is to wait and pee on them first thing in the morning after you've had a minimum of six hours of sleep. This will give you an accurate reading.

For some, dealing with stress and drinking cheap coffee go hand in hand. Now we have two things contributing to our acidity, shall we go for three? How about irregular eating patterns, alcohol, smoking, or lack of exercise? All these things can be acid forming. If you are a coffee drinker, don't panic, there is an easy way around this problem. Just keep reading my posts.

Diet can also play a part, although not in a way that most seem to understand. The good news is, the body will buffer out most acidic foods, but each time it does so it depletes vital minerals. Great if you have an abundance of minerals at your disposal, not so great if you have a bad diet that's mineral deficient. Are we there yet?

If you were paying close attention, you will have noticed that I said the kidneys and lungs help keep pH balanced. Exercise is important because it gets the lungs working. If the idea of exercise makes you cringe, then I bring good news. This following tip doesn't require you to join a gym or buy a new pair of running shoes. Check this out.

It's an exercise that isn't dependent on the weather and you can even do it while watching your favorite television show. To do this you will need a small inexpensive yoga-type trampoline. All you do is bounce on it real gentle and stop whenever you like, your cells don't care, they just like to move. The idea here is to encourage you to do whatever feels comfortable and then stop. Why?

Cells like don't like to be stagnant but they do react well to movement. Imagine a balloon half filled with water. Now in your mind's eye walk with that balloon held out in front of you. As you move, so does the water in the balloon. Now jump up and down with the balloon, this is how the energy in your cells reacts to movement. But wait there's more!

You can pick up a mini trampoline for under 50 bucks, you could even scout around online for a used one. Using a trampoline at home means you don't have to worry about people pointing at you in the gym. Using a trampoline means less jogging which cuts down on that harsh repetitive impact to the knees. And better still, you don't have to worry about stray dogs trying to bite you as you run along the street. It's a win/win.

If gentle bouncing isn't your thang, then take a walk in any direction for 30 seconds and come right back again. Excellent, you have just exercised for a whole minute, what say tomorrow we shoot for 2 minutes? The point is this, committing to an intense exercise program can be enough to talk some people out of doing it. Better to do a little at a time rather than none at all. It's easy to find reasons to stay on the couch.

If you really are a couch potato, then this next tip is just for you. Whenever you go to the store make a habit of parking your car in the far corner of the parking lot. Yup, I'm talking about the corner farthest away from the store.

Why?

For some folks, this might be the only walk they get. I'm not here to judge, I'm here to help. If that's all you can do for the day then it's important to do the best you can, not the least you can.

Walking even a short distance will get the lungs working. This, in turn, helps to contribute to the balancing of pH. If you are disabled by illness, then try to move whatever you can to get your blood pumping.

ACIDIC FOODS

Unfortunately, the standard American diet (SAD — aptly enough) is tilted toward acidity. Fast food, fried food, soda, and sugar are all acid-forming. These foods are the exact opposite of what we need to eat to be healthy. Take a look at the list below and see which of these things you consume on a regular basis. And this is by no means a complete list, but you can use it as a rule of thumb.

- meats are acidic

- vegetables are alkaline

- cola is acidic

- water is alkaline

- processed foods are acidic

- whole foods are alkaline

- cheese is acidic

- goat's milk is alkaline

- lemons are acidic outside the body

- lemons become alkalizing inside the body

Some rules tend to have exceptions, and today the exception is lemons. When a lemon is sitting on your kitchen counter, it is acidic (pH below 7). But once you eat that lemon and it is fully metabolized and becomes alkalizing (pH above 7)

Rather than inundate you with a long list of foods that are highly acidic, try to keep in mind we are simply looking to keep our body in balance.

If at any point this all gets to be too much, try to remember this simple rule of thumb. At every meal cover at least half your plate with dark leafy vegetables. Doing this one thing will help keep those excessive portion sizes under control. Greens also help detoxify, and they help alkalize. Good fats are pretty important too and I'll cover this in more detail in another post.

TEST FAIL

Now, let's see who's been paying attention. If I asked you for the pH of the body I'm sure most would quickly recall the numbers 7.35 and 7.45, and you would be wrong. The pH of the blood is 7.35 and 7.45 but the body also has a stomach, and boy is the stomach highly acidic — with good reason.

On the pH scale, the acid in the stomach is quite low, somewhere between 1 and 3 which can easily dissolve metal! But if stomach acid is strong enough to dissolve metal, why doesn't it burn through the stomach?

That's a great question but before we get to the answer lets back up a little.

Good digestion starts in the mouth. The more times you chew your food the less work your stomach has to do. Think of it this way, the better you chew, the better you poo. Once swallowed, food travels down a long tube called the esophagus. At the end of that tube is a small muscular valve that opens up just enough to allow the food to drop into a bath of stomach acid - splash!

This stomach acid (also known as hydrochloric acid, or HCL) needs to be strong enough to turn whatever we just ate into a liquid mush, this helps with absorption.

The stomach has been working this way since the beginning of time and you kinda have to marvel at the design. Once the food has been turned into a liquid mush it is ready to move onto the next stage.

But wait, there's a problem. Can you see it?

Food drops down the shoot into a bath of acid - - splosh! Food turns into liquid mush; then mush oozes out a little at a time into the small intestine, so far so good, right? Meh, not so fast…

The whole process of digestion hinges on this pivotal stage. But what if the stomach acid has become weak through illness, neglect, abuse, or simply through time?

If the acid isn't strong enough, a whole chain reaction of negative events can begin to unfold. Not least, valuable nutrients will struggle to be fully absorbed. Obviously, we need these nutrients to power and rebuild our cells.

BILLION WITH A B

Bloating, belching, flatulence, indigestion, diarrhea, and constipation are all clues that something isn't quite right with the stomach. In certain circumstances, a person with weak stomach acid may also suffer from heartburn. Wait a second, did you catch that?

But isn't heartburn treated by the million-dollar antacid industry? If only it were that simple.

If this is you, my question is this: how have years of taking antacids been working for you? Has it fixed the problem or does it just keep coming back, again and again, and again?

Obviously stomach acid is strong for a reason. Some believe that antacids only add to the problem by making already low stomach acid even lower. The stomach then strives to balance itself out, but it cannot correct the problem with a belly full of alkaline pills. Now you are caught in a constant dance with yourself. Sometimes, we need to get out of the way and let the body do the job it was designed to do.

Obviously, if you are taking a prescription antacid that is something you need to work out with your doctor to ensure this approach is right for you. While you are there, it might be worth getting tested for H-pylori which is a type of bacteria ALSO known to reduce stomach acid … just saying'.

SHIT ROLLS DOWNHILL

It's thought that a lack of stomach acid allows the valve at the end of the esophagus to open back up. This valve, also known as the lower esophageal sphincter (or LES), is a muscle that contracts much the same way the anus does. Its job is to form an important seal to keep the acid from slipping back up into the esophagus where it can cause damage and heartburn.

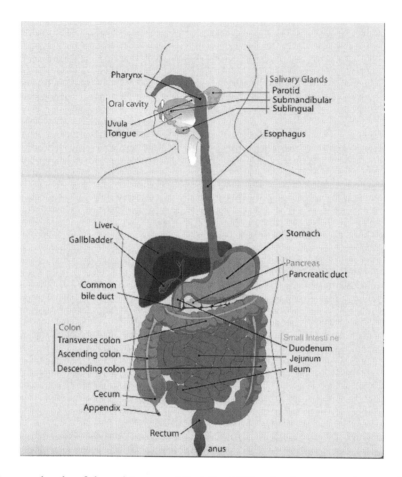

Some schools of thought suggest that the LES valve has some degree of sensitivity to the acid in the stomach. When the stomach acid is too low it may be fooled into opening back up. Hence, all those antacids aren't really helping the problem and it may be worth trying a different approach.

For now, the problem is much bigger than heartburn. Weak stomach acid has a domino effect throughout the remaining stages of digestion. The liquid mush we mentioned earlier becomes a semifluid mass of partly digested food. The fancy name for it is chyme or chymus. It's then expelled by the stomach into the duodenum.

Without wanting to confuse you with lots of fancy names let's just work with the primary rule of physics and say that all shit rolls downhill. And in this case, the liquid mush passes a whole bunch of important sensory checkpoints on the way down. These checkpoints scrutinize the quality of the mush (AKA chyme), but for now, we'll just call it liquid mush.

In theory, if the quality of the stomach acid is good, so is the quality of the liquid mush. If not, then it's a case of too bad, so sad, because when it comes to shit there really is no going backward.

Once our liquid mush enters the small intestine, enzymes are eagerly waiting to break things down even more. This can present a problem if the hydrochloric acid in the stomach is strong enough to do its job properly.

HOLD ONTO YOUR HAT, THIS IS THE TRICKY BIT

The three main enzymes the body uses to aid in digestion are amylase, protease, and lipase, but many other specialized enzymes also help in the process. Cells that line the intestines also make enzymes called maltase, sucrase, and lactase, and each is able to convert a specific type of sugar into glucose. We need these enzymes to help us absorb our nutrients.

Do we need to know all these terms as a layperson? Probably not, but I know it disturbs some people when I use terms like liquid mush and shit. - I digress ...

Two more enzymes by the names of renin and gelatinase then come into play. Renin acts on proteins in milk, converting them into smaller molecules called peptides. These are then fully digested by pepsin. I know, right? Who thinks like this?

Gelatinase digests gelatin and collagen - two large proteins in meat - into moderately-sized compounds whose digestion is then completed by pepsin, trypsin, and chymotrypsin, producing amino acids.

HERE'S THE CRITICAL BIT

If weak stomach acid allows partially undigested food to move through the digestive system, the whole delicate balance is disrupted. A domino effect occurs as the liver, gallbladder, and pancreas also pick up on the lack of acidity in the liquid mush and react accordingly. If weak acid in the stomach isn't doing its job optimally, it's a safe bet that neither is anything else.

Rather than trying to bolt the stable door after the horse has fled, it might be prudent to pay particular attention to increase stomach acid. Strong stomach acid also plays an important role in protecting us from bacteria that may be on ingested food.

SIDE NOTE

In some people, it's thought that chemotherapy can reduce stomach acid. If this is you, you may notice a sudden increase in acid reflux and this becomes all the more relevant.

To recap:

We need strong stomach acid to help us break down our foods, especially proteins. Strong stomach acid also helps kill off any harmful bacteria that may come in with food. Weak stomach acid can cause a whole host of health problems.

Before we get into this next part, let me once again stress that the following information should serve as a guide only. It cannot and should not be substituted for medical advice.

Okay, here's one way I test to see if my stomach acid is running low.

1 First thing in the morning, mix 1/4 teaspoon of baking soda in 4–6 ounces of room temp water.

2 Drink the baking soda on an empty stomach.

3 Time how long it takes before you belch.

4 If you have not belched within five minutes, stop timing.

In theory, if your stomach is producing adequate amounts of stomach acid you'll likely belch within two to three minutes. Early and repeated belching may be due to excessive stomach acid (but don't confuse these burps with small little burps from swallowing air while drinking the solution). Any belching after 3 minutes indicates a low acid level.

Because we are all uniquely different, timeframes may vary a little. This test is only a basic indicator and you might want to do more testing to determine the level of your stomach acid with your doctor. This test is a guide and not to be considered accurate enough to rule out low stomach acid. To rule out low stomach acid you will need to also try what's called the Heidelberg test or Betaine HCL challenge test.

ACV

If stomach acid is found to be too low, there are lots of ways to increase it. One is to use a supplement called Betaine HCL, (which is best taken with protein).

Another is to take a tablespoon of apple cider vinegar (ACV) 10 mins before each meal to help increase stomach acid. Simply mix the ACV in 8 oz. of room temp water and drink (for health, not taste).

If your doctor says it's okay to do so, you can raise your stomach acid by mixing one freshly squeezed lemon, 4 oz. of water, approximately three knuckles of chopped raw ginger, and a half teaspoon of sea salt.

Leave this mixture to pickle for a few days and then take a teaspoon of the mixture before meals. It's an acquired taste, but if your stomach acid is low your body may even begin to crave it. As with anything new, start with a small test dose and go slow.

If you take only one thing away from this, then let it be the value of your stomach acid. Putting our health back together is a process. And slowly, piece by piece, blog by blog, we are now bringing pieces of the puzzle into view.

So you are probably still wondering why strong stomach acid doesn't burn through the stomach. The short answer is that the stomach has a mucous membrane. It's a wall of cells that are constantly replaced; as one layer burns through, another steps in to replace it.

Finally, there's a lot crammed into this important chapter but I should also add that low stomach acid can be a factor in those suffering from hypothyroidism.

What did we learn from this?
We need the body to be slightly alkaline but the stomach needs to be quite acidic to help digest food. Stomach acid is super important to good health.

The body strives to keep our blood pH tightly regulated and it generally does an excellent job of doing so. If your body's pH is not balanced, you cannot effectively assimilate vitamins, minerals, and food supplements.

Getting gentle exercise helps regulate pH because it gets the lungs working. Committing to a short but regular exercise every day is a 100% improvement over doing nothing. You can also test your pH with litmus strips.

Homework: To help you better understand this concept take a look at a short YouTube video entitled "You thought you understood acid/alkaline diet... until you saw this!" By Peter Glidden. I think you will enjoy this one.

https://www.youtube.com/watch?v=eSuZ3fVmFMI

Chapter 12

THE IGNORANCE OF A FARMER NAMED FRED

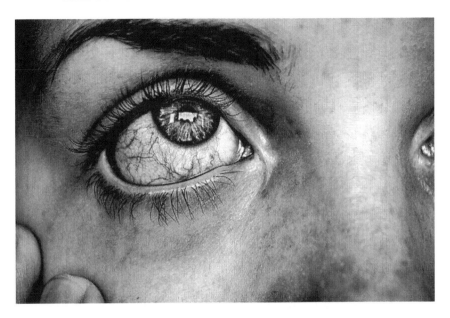

Ever wonder why today's generation is experiencing more chronic diseases, at younger ages, **than at any time in recent history?**

Growing up in the 1970s things were a little different. Back then, I don't recall a single child having food allergies, and none (as in zero) needed medication to get through the day. Our schools were just as full of bacteria and germs and yet, the number of sickly kids could be counted on one hand.

As a society, we seem to have grown accustomed to leaving the doctor's office with a prescription for a handful of pills. But still, large portions of the population remain in a state of ill health. It's no longer uncommon to see a human speeding down the road on an electric wheelchair while grasping a portable oxygen tank.

If the health of our great nation were mirrored in the animal kingdom, it would seem quite shocking. For just a moment, let's take a look at the problem from this perspective. In the following scenario, humans are played by cows and we can think of the vet as our well-meaning doctor. **Here's where the story gets interesting.**

Early one morning, a Farmer by the name of Fred sets off to feed his cows. He suddenly notices something odd and picks up his pace. On closer inspection, his cows look lifeless, tired, and show little interest in their food. The farmer eagerly rattles their food bucket in a bid to grab their attention

"Don't you want your feed today?" he asks.

A pool of large, vacant eyes stares back at him. Adding a spackle of enthusiasm to his voice he offers it a second time. "Come on girls, it's your favorite, soy and corn." (I know, right? Cows used to eat grass.)

The next morning Fred telephones the vet to explain that his cows just don't seem themselves. "They probably have CFS," says the vet.

Fred's silence prompts the vet to continue.

"I'll come to take a look this afternoon."

Fred's cows are an important commodity to him; they are his livelihood. As he anxiously waits for the vet to arrive, his mind becomes preoccupied with tracing back his steps. He knows for sure his cows weren't ill yesterday, and logically he's thinking something must have changed. But what?

Before he has time to identify the problem, the vet arrives and Fred loses his train of thought. The vet examines the whole herd and confirms that Fred's cows do indeed have a form of CFS (Cow Fatigue Syndrome).

"Is it serious?" Fred asks.

"Totally," says the vet.

Fred presses for more details, "What causes it?"

"Not sure," the vet replies.

"Well, then how do you fix it?"

"No clue."

The vet opens his brown leather medical bag and begins to inject each of the cows. By the end of the day, Fred has a bill to pay and illness continues to sweep through his herd.

For the cows, feeling ill becomes their new "normal," and by the end of summer, Fred has again noticed something very odd. A third of his cows have become obese.

Fred's wife asks, "Did you think to maybe change their feed?"

Fred reminds her that *he* is the head farmer and she is not a vet.

Again the vet is called out and this time he declares an outbreak of cow diabetes. "Not much we can do Fred, diabetes rates are climbing."

Due to the complications of advanced diabetes, some of the cows had to have their limbs amputated. But neither Fred or his wife wanted to eat steak chops for dinner.

As the autumn winds begin to blow, Fred again finds himself pressing his vet for answers. This time, the cows shiver in the cold and Fred suspects it has something to do with the town water.

"Hmm, looks like a real nasty case of Cow-pothyroidism," says the vet. Neither of the men thinks to check the water for halogens and the vet leaves with the words, "See you soon, Fred," hanging ominously in the air.

As winter rolls around, Fred's situation goes from bad to worse. Sadly, some of his cows are now dying. Without flinching, the vet delivers another blow. "Fred, I hate to tell you, but your herd now has cow cancer and eventually it will affect one out of every two cows."

The vet proceeds to cut, burn, and poison all the cancerous areas, the same way his father did it, and his father before him. As he leaves the farm, the vet thanks the farmer for his payment and tips his hat to bid the farmer good day.

A month later Fred telephones to confirm that the vet's math was indeed correct and 50% of his herd has now been wiped out. Sensing Fred's disappointment, the vet quietly utters the words, "I'm so sorry for your loss," and hangs up the phone.

Shortly before retiring to bed, Fred breaks the devastating news to his wife. "In all my years of farming I've never managed such a toxic herd." This time his wife remains silent and allows Fred's incompetence to run free. Perhaps she has been conditioned not to question.

Winter arrives, there is snow on the ground, and Fred diligently closes his books for the year. Despite heavy losses, Fred takes some comfort when he notes that his grain bill for the year was much lower than usual. Fred's wife looks over his shoulder and notes that the grain bill is only lower because Fred is using inferior grain. Despite having fewer cows to feed their vet bill was dramatically higher for the year. Once again she quietly accepts that it's not her responsibility and leaves it to the "experts" to figure out.

As winter turns to spring, Fred shrugs off his losses and adopts a positive, upbeat attitude. It's spring, the season for new life and new beginnings! But Fred's optimism is short-lived as each new calf is born. Both he and his wife know that their weakened herd is not sustainable. Eventually, everything they have worked so hard for will be lost.

Fortunately, Fred and his sickly cows are fictitious. And when we hear this story, it sounds absurd. But if we analyze the numbers from this imagined story, they are not too far from our own

We, humans, are now facing an epidemic of chronic fatigue, obesity, diabetes, autoimmune diseases, and cancer. Imagine driving through the rolling English countryside and stumbling upon a large sign that reflects human diabetes rates.

A hundred years ago, cancer was likely to affect three people out of every hundred. Today it is estimated that cancer will affect one out of every two men and one in three women (Cancer.org).

Yup, cancer is now wiping out large sections of the human population, just like Fred's cows. Despite the astonishing amounts of money being spent every day, we are actually no closer to a cure than we were a hundred years ago. How can that be right?

Over the last twelve months, just think how far technology has come. That phone in your pocket isn't just a phone, it's now a camera, a personal computer, even a live streaming video recorder! Forty years ago it would have been a struggle to fit even a calculator in your pocket! Hold that thought for a second and then ask how far we have come with cancer?

A little over a hundred years ago, aviation wasn't much more than a man flapping around with paper wings. And yet today we can jet across continents in just a few hours. In every other field, technology has moved forward at breakneck speed. But when it comes to advancements in cancer treatment, we are still using the same questionable techniques. Cancer is actually no closer to a cure than it was when the Wright brothers were doing their thing.

The twisted irony is anyone claiming to have found an inexpensive cure can expect to be ridiculed. Ensuring stagnant progress for generations to come.

It is difficult to get a man to understand something when his salary depends on his not understanding it. – Upton Sinclair

According to the American Society of Clinical Oncology (ASCO) newly approved cancer drugs can average as much as $10,000 a month. Some cut, burn and poison therapies can even top $30,000 a month!

Wait a second, are you absorbing these astronomical figures?

Sadly, waving cash at cancer offers little comfort to those whom it visits and this problem looks set to continue for another hundred years.

For now, let's stick with the cow comparison. According to the CDC's own website, it's estimated that by 2050 diabetes will affect one in four of us. Some sources believe we are already past this point. The damaging effects of diabetes on business are huge. Just in the U.S. alone, the economy takes an approximate annual hit of $245 billion through medical costs and loss of wages. The human cost of amputation is incalculable.

A worrisome uptrend in autoimmune conditions has become an omnipresent part of our bold new world. Everything from food allergies to ALS has its roots deeply embedded in the immune system. But the immune system is far from dumb, so what are we doing to make the immune system so confused that it turns against us and attacks us? There are lots of theories on this issue but today open debate and free speech aren't always welcomed.

The moral of Fred's story is clear: if we do not want to become like his cows, then we must stop acting like sheep.

What did we learn from this?

Capitalism is alive and well in the pharmaceutical industry.

Chapter 13

SUPPLEMENTS

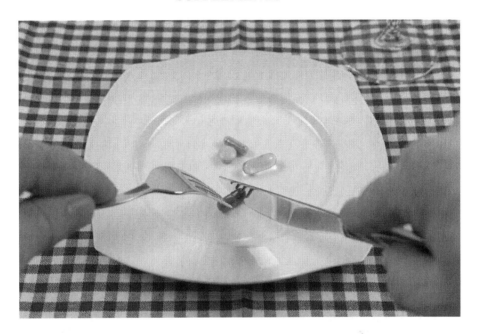

The US supplements industry is currently worth a cool $37 billion annually. For some, choosing the right supplement can be a Godsend. But for others, getting it wrong sends the whole body into an unintended tailspin. So the aim of this chapter is to help you avoid common pitfalls, and then provide workable solutions. *Ready?*

It's often said that the only difference between table salt and poison is the dose. My point is this: too much of anything is a bad thing. Popping pills without fully understanding this premise is at best foolhardy. Doing it in mega doses can be downright dangerous!

Look, we all know illness is inconvenient, and with bills to pay we sometimes make choices out of sheer panic. No work, no pay, must fix — I totally get it.

The short-term solution is to keep swallowing anything that promises relief. While the rationale for swallowing handfuls of pills is understandable, it can also become unpredictable. From the get-go, let's not make the mistake of writing a check to your body that your body cannot cash.

The body strives to be in balance and it works hard to do so. In our rush to get well, many supplements have an overwhelming effect on the body.

Why?

During times of stress or illness, the liver and kidneys are already pulling double shifts. These are the main filtering organs that process everything you swallow. This would also apply to harsh pharmaceutical drugs.

Once the liver and kidneys become overtaxed, symptoms can manifest in a whole bunch of different ways. Remember, the job of the liver and kidneys is to keep you alive by means of filtering and detoxifying. They are doing their best to keep different elements in perfect balance. Your job is to stop making this process harder.

Let's try looking at it this way.

In your mind's eye, imagine a delicate set of scales with a white feather on one tray and a small pill placed on the other tray. If the two balance each other out, then this is your body in a state of equilibrium. Today more than ever, it's much easier to disrupt this fine balancing act than it is to keep it. This then becomes the difference between feeling well or feeling ill.

Rest assured, your solutions are coming, but to fix a problem, we first have to understand it. This takes a little effort on your part, but the rewards for doing so are real. Without a clear plan, promises made by supplement companies rarely solve health problems.

Swallowing handfuls of pills to overcome illness is a bold move; if it's working for you stick with it, but in doing so it's possible to become our own worst enemy.

How so?

For some, common sense and moderation appear to have fallen out of fashion. There's a new concept in town that's completely detached from reason.

MORE IS MORE RIGHT?

We live in a fast-paced world with the widely held belief that more is more, and taking supplements in mega doses is surely a good thing, right? If only it were that easy.

In theory, EVERY supplement sounds good, but if we took every supplement that sounded good, we would soon need a suitcase to carry them all around in.

You may have diligently done your homework and read review after review before pressing that buy-now button. But keep in mind what might work for one person doesn't necessarily work for another.

That glowing review Mrs. Jones wrote for product X, Y or Z isn't going to automatically isolate you from the adverse reaction Mr. Smith had. Look, we all desperately want to swallow a magic pill that will end all our health problems, but that's not the way it works in practice.

So what's the solution?

Know that the body deserves to be in balance, so let's begin to work with it not against it. Using selective supplements that work synergistically in small groups brings much better results. However, without a firm foundation, it will rarely translate into a successful outcome.

TIPPING POINT

All things being equal, the liver and kidneys do a great job of filtering out what is harmful. But there comes a tipping point when these overtaxed organs become sluggish. As the body struggles to cope, those amazing results you were promised on the bottle will soon feel like a meandering lie. The situation then becomes far more fragile and even small doses can leave you feeling as if your health is a candle in the wind.

A good rule of thumb is this: if you aren't 100% sure of why you taking a supplement then don't buy it. Whatever it is you do buy, make yourself accountable. This can be done by simply writing down three reasons why you think supplement X, Y, or Z is going to work, and three reasons why it may not. Now we are thinking logically with our heads as opposed to acting out of fear, wishful thinking, or blind panic.

These days, it seems everybody has a product to sell you. It's super easy to be blinded by the benefits that often accompanies a product's literature. The smart thing to do is spend a little time researching the same product for its known side effects. This will help to balance out all that euphoric enthusiasm.

MULTI

In good faith, many people make an online purchase for the least expensive multivitamin in the hope that they are covering all the bases. While there is some merit to this way of thinking, it's not without problems.

Many cheap multivitamins are synthetic; they are low-quality imposters of the real thing. Often large retail stores will import supplements from abroad where it's easy to sidestep quality controls.

At this point, I'd like to stress that there are lots of good quality supplements on the market. But the misconception held by some is that "all natural" vitamins, supplements, and herbal formulas are good for you. But there's a lot more to this than meets the eye.

Inferior supplements can arrive in your medicine cabinet laced with toxic dyes. Some are even cut with talc! These types of synthetic vitamins are cheaper to make so they make more money for the company selling them.

However, buying supplements based on price will always take your health on a fruitless mission. Make no mistake, over time cheap synthetic vitamins will hurt you. They simply cannot be absorbed properly and will pull the whole body out of balance.

I can appreciate that this information might not be new to some readers but stick with me because I'll soon be going a little deeper. However, if you are a total newbie, try turning to your local health food store.

Generally speaking, small independent mom and pop type stores tend to sell better quality supplements than the big box stores. They also hold the advantage of being more knowledgeable and usually provide sound advice.

Okay, so what else do we need to know?

Vitamins fit into two groups: fat soluble or water soluble. These groups determine how vitamins are dissolved and stored in your body. Fat-soluble vitamins reside in the body's fatty tissue and liver and are used "as needed" by the body.

By contrast, water-soluble vitamins dissolve in water and are generally not stored in your body. It's worth remembering that both have the potential to cause toxicities when taken in excess.

BUT WHAT ABOUT THE DOSE?

Quality is not the only thing to worry about. How about quantity? This measurement is often a preference set by manufacturers themselves. Your health guru may tell you that you need vitamin X-Y-Z and he or she may or may not be right. But common sense should dictate that anything new that you introduce into your body should always be taken in the smallest dose first to see how you react. The term I like to use often is, start small (dose) and go slow (spread the time out).

For anyone looking for that elusive quick-fix pill, I'm aware and accept that the following sentence is about to make me about as popular as a piranha in a hotel swimming pool. Here goes nothing: supplements cannot act as a substitute for a poor diet. This is a topic we will address in more detail later, for now, let's not lose our momentum.

BE SMART AND HIT THE TARGET

If a true nutritional deficiency exists, a much smarter way is to "selectively" steer towards certain supplements. To make this point think of a rifle with a high powered telescope on the top. Now compare the accuracy of the rifle to the bluntness of a shotgun. If the two weapons were laid side by side and the goal was to hit a bullseye, might the smarter choice be accuracy?

Smaller more accurate groups of selected minerals and vitamins can work better than a broad-based multivitamin. The term for this is synergistic. This simply means certain groups of supplements work well together to produce an enhanced result. I'll be going over supplements that work synergistically in a moment, so hand tight.

By contrast, taking a multivitamin could be thought of as a shotgun approach. Now that we have all that cleared up, problem solved right? Meh, not so fast.

VITAMINS OR MINERALS?

Even if the stars aligned perfectly, you got the exact brand, the right quantity, and you even managed to accurately diagnose your own deficiency, the problem doesn't automatically end there. How so?

Vitamin supplementation fails to work optimally in a body that is lacking in trace minerals. This is super important to know because all too often the emphasis is on taking vitamins. It's minerals that make up the lion's share of your body's nutritional needs. Minerals help the body absorb vitamins, without sufficient minerals vitamins are worthless.

To some degree, the body can adapt to minor deficiencies — much like a car with a rear tail light out. The car still runs even with the broken light. Some deficiencies left to fester can become life-threatening. For example, the heart is one organ that needs a ready supply of potassium and magnesium!

GOOD NEWS

The good news is that given the correct raw materials the body (that's you) can begin to repair itself — no, seriously, the body does it all the time from the cells up.

In order to do so, the body requires approximately 90 essential nutrients. This includes 60 essential minerals, 12 Amino Acids, 16 vitamins, and 3–4 essential fatty acids.

Yup, there are more but these are considered "essential" for the simple reason that the body cannot produce them, therefore, they must be consumed. Don't worry if this seems like a lot to take in, this whole process becomes easier to understand if you just keep reading.

SCAM

In a perfect world that highly touted supplement you just ordered online would come to you at the speed of light with a guarantee that, once taken, your health will immediately spring back. Alas, the world we live in is far from perfect; sometimes we are derailed by our own lack of understanding and sometimes people make claims that are downright deceitful!

Anything man can put in a box and sell online has the potential to go wrong (or be an outright lie). So what's the solution?

It pays to buy your supplements from somebody who you know and trust. For this reason, I make a point of getting to know the names of people working in my local health food store.

When trying anything new it just makes more sense to keep it simple. If you take a handful of new supplements and something works for you, great! But how do you know which one did the trick?

On the flip side, if you feel worse after taking a handful of supplements, how will you know which caused the problem? The ideal solution is to start small and go slow.

SELF TEST

The promise of benefit is always seductive. If we find ourselves stuck in a desperate cycle of popping pills it can become a challenging habit to break. The only sure way to prove to ourselves that we have not become dependent on popping-pills is to try this easy self-test. Ready?

Try to refrain from taking ALL supplements for seven days. I know people who absolutely cannot do this and still refuse to admit they have a pill-popping problem. I also know people who have done this and have seen great improvement as their bodies come back into balance on their own.

If you have to, put all your supplements in a cardboard box and have someone save them for you. Remember, it's only a week. If this makes you feel uncomfortable, then there is a problem. Trust me on this, your body is far smarter than any Amazon seller.

If you do find yourself stuck in a loop, then the next step is to get yourself a week-to-week day planner. Write down the kind of the supplement you take, and then in brackets write down the time and the reason you take it. If you can't list the reasons, then why are you taking it?

This simple tip helps (a) serve as a record, (b) plot progress and, © keep you accountable. The latter can be quite revealing when you look back over the week. Make this process as simple as you can so it doesn't feel like a chore to do it.

Here's an example of how to keep a simple record for someone with a system that's already out of balance or easily overloaded. It's a starting point which we can always build up from later. But for now, the idea is to keep it simple so that we *don't* tax the liver/kidneys.

Tuesday 22nd November

8 am L-glutamine powder x 1 half teaspoon (gut repair)

1 pm Milk Thistle x 1 (liver detox)

3pm AHCC x 2 (immune system)

7 pm Topical DMSO (knee pain)

10 pm CBD oil (sleep)

Am I saying these are the supplements you need to take? Nope, never did say that, remember **this is just an example.** But notice how the times are spaced out? This helps us highlight what is working and what is not. If you took everything on this list at 8 am how would you work out which supplement is working and which supplement gave you a bad reaction?

Once health improves, the amounts can increase, but for now, the last thing we need to do is add to the burden of a body that's already struggling to cope. Spacing things out also prevents us from overloading the body making it easier to maintain a state of equilibrium.

As mentioned earlier, there are some supplements that work well together synergistically. But for the moment we are attempting to tackle a much bigger issue which is keeping the body in balance.

At this stage, we are trying to keep everything as simple as possible. Does L-glutamine have other benefits? Yes, but we aren't looking to write a product review here, we only need to understand our own thinking. Once this becomes a daily habit you can always expand on it by adding side notes etc.

Any supplemental gaps in between we can (and should) fill with nutrition. With the right approach, a large portion of these vitamins and minerals can be obtained from foods grown in nutrient dense soils. In simple speak, this means you aren't going to find them in processed foods.

While it might be reassuring to think a supplement that's going to take away all our problems, without a clear understanding of the subject of nutrition your health problems aren't going away any time soon. You simply can't supplement your way out of a bad diet, and with a good diet, you don't need to.

ISLAND LIVING

Think of it this way. What if you suddenly found yourself marooned on a beautiful desert island without any of your supplements or medications.

The only protein available had to be wild caught each day. The only vegetables had to be freshly picked from the land, and the only drink was fresh water or pure coconut milk — now ask yourself, how do you think your health would be a month from now?

Again, my goal is not to discourage, there are some supplements that can and do bring relief — the goal here is to help you understand the problem.

For the moment, that problem is failing to listen to your own body. Let's not forget that cheap supplements will push the kidneys and liver into working overtime. As we move forward, practical solutions will become more apparent.

I accept that recommending you buy fewer supplements isn't going to sit well with everyone. Depending on what products are being sold — it's either going to piss a few people off or it may even be the most interesting thing that they read today. Please note, I didn't decide to write this to make myself unpopular. I wrote it because it's important for anyone looking to overcome and avoid illness to know this information.

At times I might even be swimming against the popular tide here, but it beats drowning in numbers. Shall we jump in with a few supplement contradictions?

THYROID MADNESS

As Newton famously said, "For every action, there is an equal and opposite reaction." This quote serves to highlight the larger point I am striving to make which is balance is important.

It's easy to lose count of the number of contradictions that exist for every supplement out there. For example, a simple Google search reveals that iodine is essential for good thyroid health, and while this may be true, it's not the whole story.

Any thyroid that isn't functioning optimally is typically either hyperthyroid or hypothyroid. The latter being the more prevalent of the two. There is a popular school of thought that suggests that giving iodine to a person who is hypothyroid can, on occasion, be like pouring gasoline on an open flame.

Why?

A hypothyroid patient has a 90% chance of having an autoimmune condition by the name of Hashimoto's. Hashimoto's name is taken from the Japanese physician, Hakaru Hashimoto. During a flare-up, the body attacks its own thyroid.

Adding unregulated iodine either as a standalone supplement or as a mega dose multivitamin, (and to some degree iodized table salt) has the potential to magnify the problem.

The iodine contradiction is one reason why some hypothyroid patients are sent into a tailspin. Given that Hashimoto's was the first ever autoimmune condition to be discovered way back in 1934, you would have thought that manufacturers would have had ample time to understand this basic concept.

I know what you are thinking because I've had the same thought. If we know that the thyroid needs iodine, what's the solution to stop it from destroying itself?

That's a great question and the short answer lies in a selenium supplement. And here's where we begin to see the beauty of things working together synergistically. But even then it's a delicate see-saw balancing act that needs careful consideration. It's worth noting that selenium should always be taken with Vitamin E

Now we are off to the races, taking iodine (in the right dose) with selenium and Vitamin E has been shown to have an impact on thyroid-specific autoimmune disease such as Hashimoto's. Why?

Selenium significantly reduces TPO and TgAb antibodies; up to 55–86% and 35–92% respectively.

But the devil is once again in the details; too HIGH a dose of selenium can easily accelerate the problem if iodine is deficient. I know, right? Let's think before we act. The reverse is also true and each needs to remain in balance.

If either is too low (or too high) symptoms will become much worse. Both must be addressed simultaneously and in direct proportion to each other.

Sounds a little confusing right?

Even this is an overly simplified version of events, but it serves to make the point ... there is always more to supplementation than meets the eye!

Autoimmune conditions such as Hashimoto's are always a complicated business so it pays to keep an open mind. Some patients may even respond better without the use of any iodine and instead may do better by simply supporting the thyroid with supplements such as B12, Selenium, and Iron.

With thyroid problems on the rise, I'd better quickly mention that soy products can have an adverse effect on the thyroid, as can gluten. I'll write more about these another time.

If you suspect that you have any type of a thyroid issue it pays to insist that your doctor goes beyond having the standard TSH test done. The TSH test is capable of doing a great disservice to the patient because it only looks at 20% of the problem.

If you have a thyroid issue you might find the work of Dr. Izabella Wentz, Pharm. D., FASCP interesting. Dr. Izabella Wentz is a passionate, innovative, and solution-focused clinical pharmacist. What Mrs. Wentz doesn't know about the thyroid wouldn't take up any space on the back of a postage stamp.

To fully understand all these interactions and combinations it seems we might all benefit from a Ph.D. in chemistry such as Dr. Wentz has. Yet all too often we go along to the pharmacy and take the advice of the first person we can find.

VITAMIN D

Let's not limit this problem to iodine. The same argument can be put forth with just about any vitamin. Dare I say even vitamin D? While it's true that vitamin D is critical to good health, it's also worth noting that vitamin D isn't a vitamin at all, it's actually a hormone.

Vitamin D is fat soluble, which means taking too much of it can build up and cause toxicity. Taking vitamin D in pill form can be harsh on the kidneys. If you have a known vitamin D deficiency, a "sublingual" version of vitamin D is far less damaging.

Taking sublingual vitamin D simply means you allow it to dissolve slowly on the tongue which is much easier for the kidneys to process.

We should also note that vitamin D works best with calcium, the two go hand in hand and both are needed for absorption. But once again there is a little more to this story and here's where it gets a little bumpy so you might want to hold onto your hat. Ready?

If calcium is aided in absorption by vitamin D3 then K2 is also needed for it to do so effectively. Huh? But wait there's more; vitamin D is good friends with other vitamins (like vitamin A) and cooperates synergistically with minerals like magnesium and zinc.

I know, right? It seems easier to get this wrong than it is to get it right, but don't lose faith, a solution is coming.

Many of the proteins involved in vitamin A metabolism (and the receptors for both vitamins A and D) only function correctly in the presence of zinc. Surely there must be an easier way to get our vitamin D safely and in the right amount? Yes, quite often there is, and it's usually just above your head — and free…but here's the kicker. We have been conditioned over the years to cover up our living, breathing skin with sunscreen. Yet, when done sensibly, the best way to get your vitamin D is directly from the sun — in small doses.

Exposing the skin to direct sunlight for 30 mins a day in the morning can be a much safer alternative to popping vitamin D pills. As with all things, moderation is key and getting your vitamin D this way beats anything you can buy in the store by a royal mile.

Not everyone has access to sunshine year round, which makes the whole sublingual vitamin D lesson here all the more important.

DON'T DO IT

This next pitfall is one I have fallen into myself more times than I care to remember. Let's say you managed to get the correct X-Y-Z supplement and even began to feel some noticeable benefit. There is a new danger lurking in our own thinking — any guesses what it is? Top marks if you said, "Hey if one is good — two must be better, right?"

When I was ill back in 2011, I had a family to support and bills to pay. The obvious temptation was to see a small benefit and then rush forward with haste. I get it — we need to get back on our feet ASAP but the more we take the more we run the risk of increasing our chances of a setback. If ever there was a time to use the phrase, less is more, this is it. Note to self.

"It is of little consequence if flawed logic is grounded in either desperation or greed, for both will take you on a fool's errand" – James Lilley

Let's go back to that set of scales in our mind's eye. When we blindly put multiple compounds on the scale it becomes harder to keep the body in balance. This was never the way we humans were designed to digest our nutrients. What we do know, is this. The body strives for equilibrium so taking mega doses of ANYTHING makes the recovering body work harder.

So what's the solution?

If you are trying to correct a deficiency with vitamins, then food-based supplementation is generally the better way to go. Known as "whole food supplements" or "plant-based supplements," there are several good brands on the market which again, can be found in your local health food store. The golden rule is everything in moderation, for every action causes a reaction. And this reaction can sometimes involve the immune system.

IMMUNE

The immune system gets complicated which is why I'll cover in a separate post, but while we are here there is an important point I'd like you to remember. Your immune system can be stimulated or suppressed by certain supplements and herbs; this is why some people feel worse after taking supplements. Hmm, I see.

Any supplement that has the potential to cause an imbalance in the body will almost certainly rub the immune system the wrong way. And with more than a 100 autoimmune conditions primed to attack from within, creating such an imbalance can be a costly mistake to make.

Most people with an autoimmune condition spend years being misdiagnosed. At this stage let's not rule out the possibility that you could absolutely be one of those people.

Without a basic understanding of your Th1 and Th2 cells, it's never a good idea to provoke any type of immune reaction. I'll break this topic down and make easier to understand in later in my book.

BUT HOW DID WE GET HERE?

For sure our early ancestors weren't wandering around with their pockets filled with pills, so why is it that we now feel the need to supplement? The short answer to that question is relatively more straightforward than you may think.

Today, much of the commercially grown food arriving on our plate is devoid of minerals because the soil is so overworked and weak. Essentially it's been exhausted of its nutrients. Adding a handful of fertilizers to already depleted soil only adds to the problem. It's a far cry from the 90 essential nutrients our body needs to thrive.

The bottom line is this: if the foods, we choose to eat have a mineral deficiency, then we have a mineral deficiency. And from that came man's solution: mega doses of supplements! But surely this is twisted logic.

SOIL

Healthy vibrant food grown in nutrient dense soil has been shown to contain more essential minerals and it naturally repels bugs. Weaker crops, however, are more prone to infestation; they then have the added burden of being exposed to heavy chemical spraying. I know, right? Spraying the food with poison, what could possibly go wrong?

Think of soil as a bank account, if you take too much out you have to deposit some back in or the soil becomes bankrupt. This is not the way our Victorian ancestors grew food. They grew food in nutrient-dense soils that had just about every mineral you could ever need. This is common sense farming rather than simply farming for profit. Alas, as my-old-mum used to say, "Common sense isn't always that common."

Today so many of the foods we choose to eat are heavily processed and far removed from that concept. Are you getting this? It's kinda important.

Since the beginning of time, the preferred fuel to power the human body has been whole foods found in their natural state. Foods grown in nutrient dense soils are superior in every way to commercially grown foods.

Understanding supplements and the way they affect the body takes time and discipline. You should remain aware that the risk of getting it wrong is ever present, it's worth reminding that your local health store is a useful ally.

THE OTHER WAY

Taking selective supplements that work synergistically has obvious advantages, but the take-home message here is the body likes harmony. Supplements are one way to get your nutrients, but they are not the only way.

For sensitive individuals, bone broths, juicing, and even sprouting all pack a nutritional punch. For some, boosting nutritional intake this way is a safer alternative.

To those in the supplement industry, I know this idea of popping fewer pills is making me about as popular as a fart in a space suit. But before you rush to point out that I failed to include important compounds like Glutathione, Zinc, NAC, A, B, C, D, and E, yadda, yadda, yadda let me again remind you that the supplements I mention here are examples only. I'll also be writing more about which supplements are best so stay tuned.

What did we learn from this?
Controlling pain and, to some degree, suffering is as easy as popping a pill. However, this simple rationale serves only to mask symptoms and rarely gets to the root cause. The notion that you can simply swallow a pill and have all your problems go away is an appealing one, but it's fraught with complications and contradictions.

During any prolonged illness, the liver and kidneys are most likely already working overtime. This is important to remember because certain medications and supplements can force these stressed organs to work even harder

Homework: Check out this short 5-minute video, it features the insightful work of Dr. Izabella Wentz.
https://www.youtube.com/watch?v=8egFSEyav3o

Chapter 14

THE CARDBOARD BOX DIET

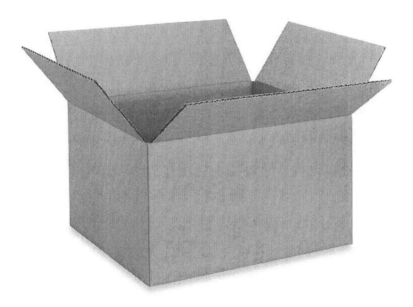

In case you missed it, food has changed more in the last 30 years than it has in the last 3000. Cows no longer eat grass; vegetables are grown in water by means of hydroponics; chickens are no longer free to roam to eat bugs; fruits are being restructured by genetic modification, and 90% of grains are being sprayed with harsh chemicals. *Gee, I wonder if any of this could have an impact on how we feel?*

To add to the problem, the vast majority of foods found on supermarket shelves are now processed. Processed "foods" might have started off as real food, but somewhere along the way, they took a wrong turn. Once foods cross over to the dark side they get to live inside a metal can, a cardboard box, or plastic wrapping along with their preservatives.

As soon as the production line has finished adding "stuff" to them, a third party turns up to collect them with the sole purpose of selling them on to you for a tidy profit. While I'm not opposed to anyone making a profit, I can't help feeling this style of production works best for the automotive industry. As you read this, keep in mind that whenever food is out of the farmers hands and into the hands of shareholders, most of what you are told about nutrition is probably wrong.

Here's where it gets tricky …

To ensures that shoppers keep coming back for more, sugar is systematically added to everything from baked beans to salad dressing, from milk to crackers. But just to keep the public on their toes, sugar goes by lots of different names. At the last count there were more than sixty ways to hide the word sugar from the label. Either way, it doesn't matter whether they call it sucrose, barley malt, dextrose, maltose rice syrup yada, yada, yada, sugar is still sugar. It's also more addictive than cocaine. No really, it's true.

To add to the problem, many of these heavily processed foods have been linked to a wide range of health problems. ADD, obesity, depression, heart disease, joint pain, and diabetes to name just a few. And while processed food is, admittedly, convenient—illness in all its many forms is certainly is not.

> The food you eat can be either the safest and most powerful form of medicine, or the slowest form of poison. – Ann Wigmore

Processed foods are high in calories but low in actual nutritional content. They won't flood your cells with key nutrients, instead, they add to your toxic burden, it's Franken food. In short, processed foods are the wrong fuel for the engine.

Here's where it gets easy …

Since the beginning of time, the human body has been designed to run on clean water and whole food. Whole foods are easy to identify because they are made from only one ingredient. Whole foods do not grow in boxes or cans. If you are still unsure, anytime you see food ask WTF? (Who's-The-Farmer?).

More than ever before in our history, people are now reacting to the foods they eat. Once our health begins to suffer, the solution is always going to be the same. We need to stop eating the wrong fuel. Am I right?

We could go around in circles all day long to make this same point sound more intelligent or complicated than it needs to be. But that heavily processed food you eat will either make you sick or keep you sick.

So here's your first golden rule: if it was made in a plant don't eat it, if it came from a plant then eat it. In the history of mankind there has never been a single recorded illness relating to a deficiency of processed foods. Seriously, never. Fortunately for us, this makes the whole transition process really quite simple.

Heavily processed food = bad.

Whole food = good.

Processed foods = more than one ingredient.

Whole foods = have only one ingredient.

As we learned earlier, processed foods are addictive, destructive and darn right deceptive. With that in mind, quitting them is easier said than done, hence we need a plan. And I just know you are going to love this!

And here's where it gets interesting ...

As any recovering alcoholic will tell you, it's far easier to avoid temptation than it is to resist it. Okay, there is no easy way to do this. What say we rip the Band-Aid off right now and get right to the solution? It's the time to take greater responsibility for your health. Ready?

Up until this point you have gotten off pretty light, but now the oven mitts are really coming off! If you want to stop making poor food choices, then I'm about to show you the absolute best way to do it.

143

First, go to the store and buy several medium-sized cardboard boxes. Fear not, the nutritional content of cardboard is of little value to us here, the boxes are needed to put your toxic food in. Once you have your boxes open them up and begin placing every single item of processed food into the box.

I know right, this guy is crazy, but keep reading anyway; I promise it gets better. As Carl Jung once said, "Show me a sane man and I will cure him for you."

Once the cardboard box is full, check to see there is a neighbor in your street who leaves a dog out to bark at night (who does that?). If so, simply gift the box to them (Or anyone else you hold a grudge against). If not, draw a skull and crossbones on it and put the damned box out for the garbage man.
I realize that this is a bold move and for some, it might be a bridge too far. If this is you, I'd like to assure you that what we have just done is absolutely critical to your success.

Here's why.

- All temptation is removed

- There are no more labels to read

- No more calories to count

- Food sensitivities, be gone

- No complicated diet to follow. Hoorah!

Still not convinced, huh?

Maybe you are fighting me on this because times are hard. If that's the case, stop and calculate the cost of the food in your cupboard. Got the figure? Perfect, now stand back and ask yourself, is that all your health is worth to you?

What do we have? Maybe a couple of hundred bucks of toxic food? I'd bet the farm that any illness would cost more in weekly medications alone. Look at it this way, if I'm right, you get your health back, if I'm wrong you lose a little money and a neighbor with the annoying barking dog gets sick. *Too bad so sad.*

If you need to save money, sacrifice something else, sell your hat or sell the cat. It's time you and your loved ones stopped sleepwalking into illness. Let this bold, decisive call to action serve as your wake up call. It's time to bite the bullet, not the biscuits.

The idea here is that we are looking for a clean slate to work with, new habits bring new results. Old habits got you into this mess! If you really want to liberate your health, put all of the processed food in the box. We both know if it remains in the house you are going to eat it.

Why is this important again?

Think of it this way, you live inside a body, if you don't take care of it, may I ask where you are going to live?

Once you clear out all that junk food, all those hidden food additives, and deceptive sugars are no longer a threat to you or to your colon (did I mention death begins in the colon?). On the flip side; once we have whole foods in the house this is what you will eat. It's a WIN-WIN.

I get it, new challenges bring resistance. And if frozen pizza has been working for you, then more power to you, if not, maybe we need to try something different.

MORE THAN JUST A PHOTO

If you need motivation find an earlier photo of yourself looking healthy, or having fun or driving a motorcycle. Once you have an image that means something to you pin it to the fridge. Obviously the photo needs to represent something bigger than your temptation, it could be a photo of your spouse or if applicable, your kiddo's.

Find something deep inside that matters more to you than a couple hundred bucks' worth of toxic food. Do this and the rest is easy.

I'm not doing this to be mean, I really do want you to succeed. Done right, this is going to work for you because this is a plan like none other you have tried. Think about it: alcoholics who successfully recover don't sit in a house full of booze.

HOW TO FAIL IN THREE STAGES

1. Keep processed food in the house.

2. Don't have a plan.

3. Repeat step one.

You might be asking, "Hey, does this also include all those condiments?" Yes, remember it's do or die, and the "do" part always seems like a much better option to me. This is a whole fresh start, with fresh food. While you are at it, send that bleached iodized salt to the box, pink Himalayan salt is better for you beyond comparison.

In case you were wondering, I've actually done this in my own life. I found it much easier to do it without thinking. Just keep putting that "food" into those cardboard boxes and this will be a breath of fresh air to your health, I promise. Now take a deep breath as we take one of those cardboard boxes and approach the fridge. I know, right? Not the fridge too!

MILK FROM A COW

Yes, obviously, this includes that block of mucus forming cheese, yes that sugar spiking organic orange juice (that's probably owned by one of the cola giants), and yes that carton of milk even if it is "fortified" with vitamin D. (D for Don't get me started.)

Now you dunnit! Milk is absolutely packed with wonderful nutrients if you happen to be a cow. Are we a cow? I think not. Humans are the only mammals on this planet that drink another mammal's milk. *I know right, what's up with that?*

But, seeing as we humans are so much smarter than the cow we have to take it a step further by taking their milk and heating it up and killing all the beneficial enzymes in the process. We then add sweeteners, and to top it all off, we stick it in a toxic BPA plastic container for its 1500 mile ride to the store. It's only use now is to make the mind boggle … and the food manufacturers have the audacity to call this healthy!

If you want your health back you have to fight for it, so yes, this step is important and we don't want you to be even an eenie-weenie little bit tempted.

If you simply can't throw food out, then seal the box and have someone save it for you for thirty days. Your fridge should now look just like it did the day you bought it. Empty!

PUSH BACK FROM FAMILY MEMBERS

If you happen to share a fridge, I accept this step may be more challenging, so you now have two options for you. First, get the whole family on board, maybe even get them to read this (hello family member) this way everyone knows where you are coming from. Getting family members on board would be an ideal solution. It wouldn't kill them to eat healthy, whereas eating toxic food certainly might!

However, if you are feeling a certain amount of pushback, or your family members refuse to cooperate, I have a simple fix. Simply unplug the freezer for a few hours and say, "Hey guys, we lost power and I had no choice but to throw all the food out!" The point is this: if you are determined, you will find a way, if not you will find an excuse.
Okay, almost there, just one last important thing to know in advance. Whenever you set about to change your life, people will inadvertently attempt to derail your attempts. It's just the way it is.

As sure as night follows day, the second you remove all temptation from your home someone is going to knock on your door and offer you cake.

Knowing that people are going to try to tempt you in advance gives the power back to you. This power comes from within and you should not count on the support of others for your success. Remember the rule. The cake is coming, but do not accept the cake.

At this stage, you may be forgiven for saying, "Gee, after I do all this cleaning out, what the heck am I going to eat?" I'm so glad you asked. Stay tuned because it's actually so simple even a fat burning caveman could do it.

What did we learn from this?
When faced with illness treat anything that comes in a box, a can, or a packet with suspicion. Removing all processed foods from your cupboards not only removes temptation it takes all the guesswork away.

Homework: Pick up some cardboard packing boxes...you know the drill.

Chapter 15

HIT THE RESET BUTTON

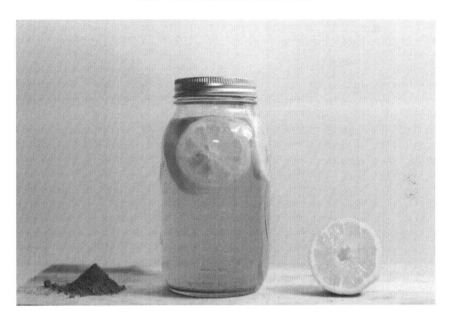

Your body is smart. Ever notice the first thing it does when we become ill? It shuts itself down, forcing us to rest. Next, we lose our appetite. *Why?*

Digesting food is a labor-intensive process taking valuable energy away from a body that's trying to heal. Think about it, we bombard our digestive system with foods even the bugs won't eat. Throw into the mix handfuls of pills, and additives with unpronounceable names. Now we are really asking our digestive system to go to work!

I wonder, how would you feel if your boss pushed you this hard and then said you couldn't take the weekend off. Perhaps tired, depressed, lethargic, or even chronically fatigued? Hmm, I see.

Taking an occasional break from food gives the digestive system a chance to regroup and regenerate itself. It's also an effective way to clean out toxins while increasing energy and boosting mental clarity. The name for this is intermittent fasting. But this isn't a new idea, it's actually a tried and tested principle that dates back to pre-biblical times.

I know what you are thinking because I thought it too. Nobody wants to go hungry, am I right? The good news is there's a trick to doing this so that you don't feel hungry.

Maybe you missed it but Jared Leto found it, so did Gwyneth Paltrow, Anne Hathaway, and Beyoncé to name but a few. If done right, this technique can be like hitting the reset button to your health!

Okay, let's get down to the money part. Here it comes ....

The following information is actually available to you free of charge. The raw materials required can be found in every grocery store. Better still, this will cost you less than the price of your daily coffee, Hoorah!

Okay, there is one small catch, but I'll get to that in a moment. On the plus side, if you get this right, the rewards can be nothing short of astounding. Drum roll, please!

Welcome to THE MASTER-CLEANSE!

The Master-Cleanse is the brainchild of Stanley Burroughs. Over the years it's been successfully completed by more people than you can shake a hairy stick at. It remains popular today (even with the Hollywood set) because it works really, really well. Here's why.

The Master-Cleanse helps to clean out the liver and kidneys, while at the same time giving the digestive system time to repair. Once the burden of food sensitivities is lifted from the body, batteries are quickly recharged and key nutrients flow into the cells. Stanley Burroughs believed that a toxic body that is not eliminating properly is the root of all illness.

That said, to pull this off it takes a disciplined mindset, (or simply a strong desire to get well). It may also take a couple of attempts to get the hang of it. For those who do complete it, they will begin to crave clean foods over junk foods, no question about it.

I've actually done the Master-Cleanse several times and found it's a great tool to have in the toolbox. But the Master-Cleanse isn't recommended for anyone taking medications because the two simply don't mix. If this is you, keep reading because there's still a lot of solid information to be learned here. And who knows? Perhaps down the road, your circumstances may even change. For now, it's important to work with your own doctor and try to scale down any medication gradually over time. That would be the smart thing to do.

In 1941 Mr. Stanley Burroughs published a small booklet on the "Master Cleanse" which is available as a free download online. It's well-written and very easy to understand. A hard copy is still in print and can be found on Amazon.com. (Details in today's homework section.)

So my goal here isn't to take away from someone else's book. It's to give you a few of my own helpful tips on how to do the Master-Cleanse successfully. The exact protocol is always better coming directly from the source.

OMG, SALT?

There are two parts to the Master-Cleanse, the first is the salt-water-flush (say what now?) first thing in the morning. If you can get your head around that, the rest is a stroll in the park. Why do we need part 1?

Well, over the years the digestive system can become impacted with rancid fats, proteins, and fecal matter. I know, right? Gross. But once you remove this thick slimy coating digestion improves along with health. The salt-water-flush (huh?) helps facilitate digestion by cleaning the entire digestive system from top to bottom.

You may have heard of colonic irrigation which has become a recent trend that's not without merit. But for my money, the salt-water-flush (geez, he just keeps saying it) does the job much better. Not least, because it works in the correct direction, from the top down. Colonic irrigation works from the bottom up (intended pun).

The other advantage of the Master-Cleanse is it can also be done in the comfort of your home. And for a fraction of the cost of colonic irrigation.

The first attempt at a salt-water-flush (he said it again) may be a little uncomfortable as all the junk in the trunk becomes dislodged. It might take a couple of attempts to get things moving so hang in there. Once things get kick-started it will move through much easier and faster next time. If digestion has been a problem for you in the past, then this step is going to be more challenging. Drinking a Smooth-Move tea at night may prove helpful.

If you don't manage to "flush" the first time, you may need to check that you have the correct dose of salt before trying to drink more. There, I said it. Busted. Yup, it's true, the first part of the master cleanse includes drinking salt water in the morning on an empty stomach. I know right, but keep reading, there is an upside coming.

I know we have all been conditioned to think salt is bad for us, but there is actually a lot of science behind this cleanse. If you have unanswered questions about the salt water flush, there are lots of YouTube clips on the topic.

Done right, (as per the exact Stanley Burroughs protocol), the salt-water-flush isn't going to be in your system for very long (if you catch my drift). The trick is to give yourself a dedicated hour in the morning and a definite need to stay close to a bathroom—so plan ahead. Once the flush is complete, you can go about your day, as usual, feeling lighter and refreshed.

Psychologically you need to be up for this. When I was at my most ill, I reached the point where I no longer cared what anything tasted (or looked) like so long as it gave positive results. For me, this step, along with several others, brought results.

Before we move onto part 2, it's important to note that you CANNOT under any circumstances use regular table salt. Refer to the Stanley Burrows protocol for full details.

PART 2

The second part of the Master-Cleanse is actually quite pleasant. It's another drink but this time it tastes much better than it sounds. No really. It also does a great job at keeping hunger at bay.

The Master-Cleanse drink has three key ingredients making it super easy to follow. They should be made fresh each day using the following: organic lemons, grade B maple syrup, and a pinch of cayenne pepper. Any time you manage to try the salt-water-flush (oh come on) you will find you crave the lemons.

Depending on personal preference, you can reduce the amount of maple syrup in each drink. But you really can't skimp on the quality of these three ingredients which are critical for success. Keep in mind, the additional cost of going organic is relatively easy to justify because you aren't buying food. If you stop and do the math, buying coffee would actually cost you more over the course of a week.

Grade B maple syrup is the preferred choice because it's produced later in the season. This makes it's darker and more maple flavored and it's also higher in minerals than standard maple syrup. In some areas, the term "Grade B" has been replaced with the term "Grade A Very Dark" or "Extra Dark." This isn't done to confuse people; it's done to comply with new international standards for labeling maple syrup.

The key to succeeding with the master cleanse is preparation. Have everything you need ahead of time because running out of lemons is a great excuse to quit halfway through. Mix up a batch of drinks before you leave the house and take them with you in a small cooler.

HOW LONG?

The Master-Cleanse can last however long you like. It's important to listen to your own body and only do what feels right. Typically, the Master-Cleanse can last for 10 days. Depending on your levels of toxicity, you may hit a few bumps on the way. The first four days can be challenging but once you get past that point your body switches into fat burning mode. Boomshakalaka! Once that happens, fasting gets so much easier and your thoughts become crystal clear.

Okay, here's how to make the juice.

Use a 16oz glass mason jar and fill it with clean, room temperature water (it's easier on digestion). Add three tablespoons of freshly squeezed lemon juice into the glass jar, bonus points for using organic lemons. Then add one teaspoon of maple syrup and a pinch of cayenne pepper to taste. Maple syrup is lower on the glycemic index score than regular cane sugar. It's also got a certain antioxidant value to it, which regular sugar does not. If you are trying to get into ketosis (more on this later) you could reduce the amount of maple syrup.

The pinch of cayenne helps with digestion, boosts metabolism, and gives detox support. When you mix these three key ingredients together it has a surprisingly nice kick to it.

Before jumping in with both feet, you can try this drink for a few days as a replacement for breakfast and see how you do. Don't be surprised if it holds you over as much as any breakfast meal would. For the rest of the day eat as normal. The idea here is to build confidence that you can do this for longer periods.

When you feel ready, try cranking it up a little. Maybe the next day instead of making just one drink for breakfast try making two and see if you can through lunch time until dinner. As your confidence grows, keep stretching out the time until you can do a full day, and so on.

My wife doesn't care too much for the cayenne taste so she takes less, but I actually like it. She also prefers more maple syrup and I prefer less. My point? Find what works for you.

The brilliant part of the Master-Cleanse is the healing power of the lemons. Here's why:

- Room temp lemon water encourages the production of bile

- It's a great source of citric acid, potassium, calcium, phosphorus, and magnesium

- Despite being acidic, lemons help keep your pH balance in check

- Lemons are an excellent and rich source of vitamin C

- Lemon water helps to detoxify the liver and kidneys

- Lemons contain pectin fiber, which serves as a powerful antibacterial

- Gives the body a break from food sensitivities

The last bullet point is especially helpful. Food sensitivities can result in anything from debilitating migraines to chronic fatigue.

To add to the complication, there is sometimes a disconnect between the food and the time it takes to react to it. Not everyone with a food sensitivity turns blue and immediately rolls around on the floor. The master cleanse allows us to spot food sensitivities as food is gradually reintroduced.

Once food sensitivities are removed from the body, good things begin to happen. Any time we lift the burden, it helps the body heal.

The master cleanse has been tried and tested by thousands of people with positive results. That said, whenever toxins are removed from the body, it's always best to do it slowly. The more toxic your liver is, the slower you will want to go. Being aware of this ahead of time gives you ample opportunity to find a coping strategy.

TIPS FOR ENDING A 10-DAY FAST

The reward for getting to this point is food will now smell and taste very different. Your body will seek out clean food. However, it's important to ease yourself back into eating solid food to avoid the risk of digestive upsets. Stanley Burroughs recommends ending the fast in the following way.

Day 1—At the end of the 10-day fast, slowly sip on an 8 oz. glass of freshly squeezed organic orange juice. You can also dilute the juice with clean/filtered water.

Slowly drinking orange juice prepares the digestive system for regular food, doing this step right will help give digestion a blank slate to work up from. Not too much orange juice mind you; we don't want to flood the body with a form of liquid sugar. And after ten days of fasting, this is something to be mindful of.

Day 2—The next morning again gently sip on a glass of freshly squeezed organic orange juice, adding extra water if needed. In the afternoon begin preparing a homemade vegetable soup. This doesn't have to be bland in anyway shape or form, you can add celery, carrot, onion, kale, potato, greens, okra, tomato, squash, zucchini, green peppers, yadda, yadda, yadda. But DO NOT add any meat. At least for now.

Cut the vegetables into small pieces to aid digestion. Add sea salt for taste and let the soup simmer. Once cooked, first try sipping a cup of the broth because it's loaded with nutrients and will further aid in digestion. Then take the soup as your first evening meal.

trust me, after 10 days of fasting, this will be the best-tasting soup you've ever had! Store the remaining soup in the fridge for tomorrow. Don't waste all your hard work by cramming bread and crackers back into your diet.

Day 3—Drink a small amount of fresh-squeezed orange juice again in the morning, not too much now, just enough to aid digestion. At lunchtime have the vegetable soup leftover from the previous day. For your evening meal, use any leftover vegetables to make a salad.

Keeping things simple will really help you to highlight any sensitivities. If you want to do this, it's worth doing right, stay away from the big four: bread, milk, cheese, and eggs.

Days 4—Congratulations, you are almost there. Continue to ease back into eating clean foods such as soups, salads, freshly sprouted seeds, and a small amount of fruit.

Over the next few days, slowly begin adding in grass-fed meats. As you slowly introduce solid foods back into your diet, be aware of how they make you feel. Keeping a food journal may prove helpful.

The master cleanse is an ideal way to clean up your diet after being on the road or overindulging during the holidays. With that in mind, I'd like to challenge you to make a habit of doing this once a year as part of your annual spring cleaning.

Ironically, as I end this I noticed a movie has recently been made about the Master-Cleanse. It stars Kyle Gallner, Anjelica Huston, and Anna Friel. If you have the ability not to take yourself too seriously, this might be something worth taking a look at.

What did we learn from this?
The master cleanse helps the body shed toxins while flooding the body with key nutrients. It also gives the digestive system a chance to rest and repair.

The first four days of any cleanse can be the most challenging; after that, your body enters a fat burning mode and your thinking will naturally become much clearer. The Master-Cleanse might not be for everyone, but for some, it can help to fix a multitude of sins in one swoop.

Homework: Check out "The Master Cleanse" by Mr. Stanley Burroughs. It's available as a free download or you can purchase a hard copy through Amazon (ISBN 9781607966074)

Author note

Like what you read so far? If so, a short review from you would be awesome.

Many Thanks

Chapter 16

TOXIC OVERLOAD

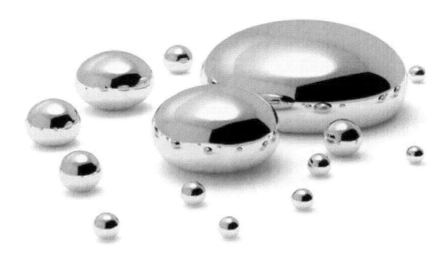

At some point, your body will come into direct contact with a toxic heavy metal, no question about it. How well you handle that exposure depends on the following three things.

1. The substance

2. The amount of time spend coming into contact with it

3. Your ability to detoxify it

Heavy metals are any relatively dense metal with an affinity for pushing good health off the edge of a cliff. **In short, heavy metals are to you what kryptonite is to Superman.** Here's why…

In 1974, The World Health Organization reported that 82% of all chronic degenerative disease was caused by toxic metal poisoning. And yet, when we look at the Earth's crust as a whole, heavy metals were once relatively scarce. *Ever wonder how we got to this point?*

The link between heavy metals and serious health problems can be traced back to the industrial revolution. Back then, manufacturing techniques allowed metals to seep into our waterways, our soil, and the air we breathe.

Today, corporations around the world continue to add toxic materials to our daily products. It's now become commonplace to find lead in lipstick, arsenic in wood preserver, cadmium in batteries, aluminum in deodorant, and the list goes on and on and on.

Trace amounts of heavy metals now turn up in fruit juice, prescription medications, health supplements, and even baby formula! As a result, getting metals into the body is the easy part. As for getting them out again? Well, that's a little trickier.

A lot can be said for eating healthy, but no amount of kale soup is going to chelate heavy metals (organic food is tested for pesticides, *not* heavy metals).

The good news is, with the right approach, your body is capable of shedding these toxic substances. **In the process, energy soars, brain fog lifts, and a peaceful night's sleep becomes achievable.** (More on this later).

That said, unraveling the damage caused by heavy metals is a process. Not least because symptoms present themselves in so many different forms. Once we have one health-destroying heavy metal floating around inside us the risk of accumulating another increase.

When the body deals with heavy metals, it used the liver, kidneys, lungs, GI tract, and skin as filters. When the burden becomes too great, (or too frequent), these delicate organs will become less effective. But there's a bigger problem lurking, *can you see it?*

The brain doesn't have a filter; it has a protective barrier around it. It's there to prevent toxins from entering. But heavy metals such as lead, mercury, and aluminum are too powerful and cross that barrier with ease.

Once inside the brain, the pituitary is left exposed. This small gland is only about the size of a pea but it's a critical player in your endocrine system.

Why?

The pituitary gland produces melatonin. Melatonin is a wonderful hormone that regulates sleep-wake cycles. Without sleep, the brain doesn't get a chance to repair and detoxify itself. New evidence suggests that as we sleep the brain shrinks allowing spinal fluid to flood. It's the equivalent of a cleanup crew coming into clean the store after hours.

But heavy metals such as mercury, aluminum, and lead unnaturally stimulate the pituitary. This might explain why some folks feel "tired and wired" at bedtime. It can feel like the mind "chatter" just won't shut off.

The pituitary gland also plays a key role in our intuition. When our intuition is off we lose the ability to sense when something is immediately and instinctively wrong. Perhaps here we see the birth pangs of mental anguish and anxiety.

Let's explore this a little.

When a heavy metal is present in the brain rational thinking becomes an unachievable skill. At best, foggy thinking becomes the new norm; at worst a person is capable of lashing out in either anger or frustration. Perhaps both are consequences of a mind that is slowly being poisoned.

Clearly, the human mind cannot cope with heavy metal exposure. I'm sure many have heard the term "mad as a hatter". A reference to English hat makers who, not so long ago, used heavy metals as part of their hat-making process. These craftsmen were well known for their irrational outbursts and depressive bouts. Symptoms were attributed to the Mercury used in finishing top hats. Once the mercury seeped into the bloodstream it was only a matter of time before it crossed the blood-brain barrier.

But mercury isn't the only heavy metal to causes mental problems. Lead is another neurotoxin also associated with major depression, reduced IQ, and anxiety disorders.

It was once speculated that the fall of the mighty Roman Empire was due in part to the introduction of lead plumbing.

Because of their high degree of toxicity, arsenic, cadmium, chromium, lead, and mercury all play a significant role in mental health, although this is by no means a complete list. Bottom line: when the burden of heavy metals overwhelms the body's ability to detoxify them, health problems begin to intensify.

And yet, developing countries continue to release toxins into the atmosphere by the ton. Once these volatile poisons are whipped up into the airstream it's anybody's guess where they will land.

THE WEAKEST LINK

Unfortunately, it's not just the brain that's exposed. Toxic heavy metals can settle just about anywhere in the body. Be it in the thyroid, prostate, heart, muscle, or even bone. When heavy metals settle in their new home they do a first-class job of messing with body chemistry.

How so?

Heavy metals are masters of disruption and will often disrupt essential minerals. As an example, thallium mimics potassium which can affect nerves and cardiovascular system. Cadmium is known to displace zinc, and lead is so chemically similar to calcium it leaches into the bones. This process happens faster in a body that is deficient in minerals.

Minerals help to perform functions necessary for life. The five major minerals in the human body are calcium, phosphorus, potassium, sodium, and magnesium. These minerals were once found in abundance in the foods we ate. Unfortunately, we now live in a world where food is grown for profit, not mineral content.

At this point, it's prudent to mention that a decrease in minerals can happen gradually over time. This can cause a real disconnect between exposure and sickness the insidious build-up of heavy metals.

WHEN SILVER BECOMES MERCURY

In the past, I've successfully dealt with my own exposure to mercury, arsenic, uranium, and lead. Hence I have a keen interest in the topic. This led me to the work of one of one of the world's leading experts, Dr. Chris Shade, Ph.D.

As Dr. Shade pointed out, "silver" dental fillings contain an element of mercury. Once they become an integral part of the tooth, mercury vapors begin to trickle down into the rest of the body. This happens around the clock, 365 days a year.

Over time this buildup compounds and in the process causes a multitude of health problems. Removal of silver fillings is the only way to prevent further exposure. However, in the wrong hands, removal can add to the problem. (Been there done that, and now have the damned tooth extraction to prove it). Working with an educated dentist who fully understands the dangers is critical. Sadly, most don't.

Heavy metals experts all agree that these types of fillings should have been banned years ago. Despite a mountain of evidence alerting dentists to the obvious dangers, some (through either ignorance or arrogance) continue putting "silver" fillings into the mouths of children. The idiotic argument often put forward is that metal fillings are stronger, sheesh, thanks for nothing.

Unfortunately, heavy metals aren't confined to teeth. It should come as no surprise that some of the highest readings for heavy metals are found in our waterways. As such, methylmercury is routinely found in many fish supplies. The higher up the food chain you go the higher the concentration of mercury. Shark, Swordfish, King Mackerel, and Tilefish are all notoriously contaminated. Smaller fish like sardines would be a better choice. Not only are they lower in the food chain they also contain selenium. This can have a protective effect on any potential mercury exposure. It's a WIN/WIN for fish eaters.

If you aren't a fish eater, be sure to remain vigilant if you supplement with fish oils. Some of the more reputable sellers like Nordic Naturals offer third-party testing. Third party testing ensures that someone who is perceived to be independent checks the fish for excessive levels of mercury.

MASTERS OF DISRUPTION

The havoc heavy metals cause is without limits. To understand why we need to dig a little into the chemistry. Don't let this part phase you in any way, by the time we end this chapter you will have a much clear understanding. *Ready?*

Remember, what heavy metals do best is disrupt, it's their party piece. This includes messing up enzyme activity. Enzymes help regulate different processes in the body. They also make certain chemical reactions happen. Whenever a cell needs something done in a hurry it uses enzymes to speed up chemical reactions.

Enzymes are special types of proteins. Like all proteins, they are made from strings of amino acids. Why is this important to know?

Inside the amino acid, cysteine group is the sulfhydryl group. Sulfhydryl groups are great at moving electrons around and holding the good metals in place like copper and zinc. Unfortunately, the thing that also likes to link up with sulfhydryl groups is our old friend mercury. Once mercury gets attached, it displaces the copper or the zinc that was supposed to be there.

Zinc is required for the catalytic activity of more than 300 enzymes; it's involved in the synthesis and metabolism of carbohydrates, fats, proteins, nucleic acids, and other micronutrients.

But it doesn't stop there.

Copper and zinc are a team that likes to work together. Copper is important for a healthy heart, bones, and brain development. Zinc is an immune-system booster that helps the body stay healthy. But everything it's a delicate balancing act. Copper and zinc have an interesting relationship. The intake of one causes the other to decrease in the body.

A healthy balance between the two is critically important to prevent a buildup of toxicity in the body. Throw in the mix a destructive heavy metal and the fine balance soon becomes unglued.

Are we there yet?

Copper and zinc are important **but so are all the other minerals.** The heart needs calcium, magnesium, and potassium or it simply won't pump smoothly. Heavy metals mimic essential minerals but ultimately they are preventing minerals from doing their job. When that happens, heavy metals have the potential to send every system in the body out of balance. To add to the problem, without minerals, vitamins cannot be absorbed.

Now, let's shift back to the brain. Can you imagine the complexity of the problem once heavy metals cross the blood-brain barrier and enter the mind? Can we expect to see a little brain fog? I think so.

FIGHTING FATIGUE?

Alas, our problems don't stop with a foggy brain; once heavy metals disrupt enzyme production essential nutrients are blocked from reaching the mitochondria.

Mitochondria are the tiny powerhouses inside the cell. Think of them as the battery inside your watch, when the battery runs down the watch slowly runs down. Whenever mitochondria take a hit so does your energy. Just for good measure, we now experience chronic or debilitating fatigue.

By now you should be realizing that heavy metals are not only destructive; they can be very difficult to remove. Here's what you need to remember.

Whenever an attempt is made to remove heavy metals, the golden rule is don't be greedy. This simply means that chelation (removal of metals) needs to be done slowly. Detoxification is a marathon race, not a sprint. Any attempt to do this too quickly will cause you to crash and burn. Trust me, I've been there and you don't want that.

Without a clear plan, heavy metals can be an extremely complicated riddle to solve. With that in mind, I'm currently working towards releasing a separate book that delves deeper into this fascinating subject. In it, I'll show you how to test for heavy metal toxicity. I'll also share some effective detoxification protocols that you can try from home. Others. you may need to work with a health care professional.

For now, I'd like to leave you with three tips to help reduce your toxic burden. **Each is highly effective, noninvasive, and easy to.**

Whenever an attempt is made to remove heavy metals, the golden rule is don't be greedy. This simply means that chelation (removal of metals) needs to be done slowly. Detoxification is a marathon race, not a sprint.

With that in mind, I'll share three noninvasive, detoxification protocols you can try from home. Others. you may need to work with a health care professional.

TIP #1

As I'm sure many already know, the liver is the bodies main detoxification organ. So this first tip is intended to support the liver. Once we get this bad boy fired up good things happen!

To do this we need only three things. A mason jar, celery, and access to a juicer.

Each morning drink 16 ounces of celery juice on an empty stomach. Remember, we are drinking this for health, not taste. Don't be over complicating things by adding in more ingredients. No apples, no lemon, no ginger, no spinach, nada, zilch, zero. It simply won't work as well and any intended benefit will be lost.

For the first few days, you might not feel the difference but as the days roll on don't be surprised if your mood improves and you begin to feel brighter and lighter. Among other things, celery juice is teeming with powerful anti-inflammatory properties. Inflammation, is the driving factor behind a wide range of "mysterious" illnesses.

(Tip of the hat to Anthony William's for bringing this tip into the mainstream).

TIP #2

There's a mountain of evidence to show that infrared saunas are one of the safest, yet most effective ways to remove heavy metals. As an added bonus, light rays penetrate several inches in the skin, fat, and muscles of your body. This also helps to improve energy levels via the mitochondria which respond positively to this type of light. *No really, it's true.*

For most of us, buying an infrared sauna isn't an affordable option. The good news is your local gym probably already has a sauna. Bonus points if it's infrared! If not, try calling around.

TIP #3

Moving along nicely let's put into a place our first binder. Binders help to soak up heavy metals. There are lots of different types out there but Pectasol-C supports a healthy immune system as well as aiding gentle detoxification.

Unlike other binders (such as activated charcoal) Pectasol-C doesn't chelate (remove) important minerals. Pectasol-C is a form of modified citrus pectin. It promotes safe detoxification as well as encouraging healthy cell growth and proliferation.

What did we learn from this?

Coming into contact with heavy metals is now a daily occurrence. When the burden becomes too great on the body, heavy metals can present a wide range of serious health problems. Heavy metals also disrupt enzymes and block essential minerals.

It's advisable to get yourself tested and find an informed health professional to work with.

Homework: For more information relating to heavy metals check out a lady by the name of Wendy Myers at https://myersdetox.com/ Wendy has a great deal of insight and a genuine passion for this important topic.

Chapter 17

STAY OFF THE SUGAR TRAIN

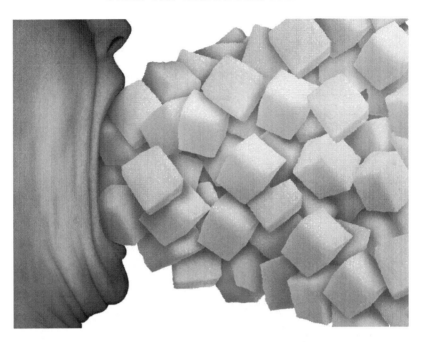

Earlier this week I attempted to move at speed through my local supermarket. My flow was soon interrupted by a six-foot wall of soda stacked on pallets. One sugar spike side-stepped, and I'm immediately presented with another. Brightly colored cakes, cookies, and pastries, all neatly lined up to whisper sweet nothings in my ear.

Full speed ahead and I can't help but notice there's another isle that resembles a well-stocked candy store. Making a hard left, I cruise past the boxed cereals, yup, all heavily laced with more sugar.

Up past the freezer section and I'm forced to do mental combat with the ice cream and popsicles peddlers. Finally, I find what I'm looking for and head to the checkout. As I stand in line I can't help but notice there's a glass-doored refrigerator to my right. Its another sugar trap bursting at the seams with soda and fruit juice. To my left, it's a full-on sales pitch from the bubble gum and candy reps.

As I shuffle forward the checkout lady glances up at me and smiles. She then asks if I'd like to donate a dollar to diabetes research? I know, right? You can't make this stuff up!

First, we have to give credit where it's due. Supermarkets really do know how to sell us a product. All too often we don't even realize that we are being sold to!

Supermarket floor plans are purposefully arranged to make us go wherever they want us to go with the sole intention of getting us to part with hard cash. Colors and labels are arranged not by chance but in a calculated bid to grab our attention. The longer we are in the store the more we are unwittingly influenced to buy things we didn't know we needed. Ever go into a store for lettuce and leave with a pair of socks?

Make no mistake, the food industry is hugely profitable, as such it can afford to run marketing campaigns at peak meal times. This ensures that most of our dietary information comes from the people we should trust the least: those with a product to sell us!

At best this information is a conflict of interest, at worst, it's a form of manipulation. I'm sure we've all heard the classics "Grains fortified with vitamins for a healthy heart" or "Low fat to stop you from getting fat"

The timing of these commercials is ultra slick and their effectiveness can stretch across generations. I suspect if we dug a little deeper, we'd soon learn that much of the nutritional advice we own today was handed down to us by our well-meaning parents. "Drink your milk up, it's good for bones" If only it were that easy.

Let's strive to keep this simple. There are only two types of foods of interest to us, those foods that keep us healthy and those foods that keep us sick.

Here's the rub.

Ask most people if they eat healthily and you will usually get this response, "Yup, I eat fairly healthy." Now we see the problem for what it is. A fairly healthy diet is a perception or a belief system that's built on the back of misinformation.

Few people think, hmm, best I nip myself down to the shop and load up on some toxic anti-nutrients and sugar. Nope, that idea is often gifted to us by the people selling us our food in the form of subliminal advertising.

So this idea that we have "a fairly good diet" is a dangerous one. Those in the first flush of youth may get away with it for a while. But the longer we allow ourselves to listen to this mainstream hogwash the sicker we all become.

To be clear, the food industry is in business to make a profit. There's nothing wrong with making a profit especially if it creates "meaningful" employment. But it's important to understand the laws of business are simple. Cheap and quality cannot coexist in the same product.

Ever notice how supermarkets are constantly trying to undercut their competition? On the surface, this might seem like a good deal for the consumer, but from a health point of view, it a race to the bottom. Maybe it's time we stopped asking why healthy food is so expensive and start asking why junk food is so cheap?

Discount supermarkets are missing out on a huge opportunity. A strong undercurrent of better-informed consumers is now walking through their doors every day. People are waking up to the idea that sugar and preservatives solve one problem, but cause another of greater magnitude.

Alas, rather than take the bold move to sell quality rather than price, supermarkets are hell-bent on trying to trick us into buying more of the wrong foods. In a classic bait and switch routine, we are encouraged to count calories rather than look at nutritional content. Such supermarket trickery is well planned and executed with seamless perfection.

No?

It might surprise you to know that the food industry employs teams of highly paid psychologists. Whoa! Why would a supermarket want to have someone that studies human emotions and behavior on the payroll?

The answer to that question is simple: supermarkets are keen to find the best way to tap into your brain-reward-system. The brain-reward-system is well documented and involves several parts of the brain. Once they have this mapped out they can hack into your spending habits.

THE BRAIN REWARD SYSTEM

Before time became a thing, the reward system was hardwired into your brain as a way to help you survive. Back then, it wasn't possible to find sweet tasting fruit that was out of season. The reward for finding certain foods that tasted of salt, fat, and sugar was an instant hit of dopamine.

Today we can pick up strawberries in the dead of winter and dopamine still rewards us with a hit of pleasure. But there's a problem, can you see it?

Whenever the brain-reward-system kicks in it changes brain chemistry in a way that drives people to over-consume. This is good news for food industry profits, but not so good for anyone trying to break the junk food cycle. Hence overindulgence has an addictive quality to it. It's also the reason why you can't eat just one cookie.

The word "addiction" is derived from a Latin term for "enslaved by" or "bound to." Anyone struggling to overcome a sugar addiction will understand the challenge this brings. According to USDA Economic Research Service, the average child under twelve is now addicted to consuming, on average, forty-nine pounds of sugar per year!

CHILDREN GETTING HIT HARD

As adults, we get to make our own decisions and live by them. But children are getting a sugar hit from all angles. Who's going to say no to birthday cake, Halloween candy, or the ice cream truck on a hot day?

Kids are then systematically targeted by TV commercials that encourage them to eat sugary cereals for breakfast. To add to the problem well-meaning family members often have a steady supply of sugary treats on hand. Hey, thanks for the cavities, Grandma.

You might be wondering how adding sugar to the food supply (as a way to increase profits) is even legal. But with one in four kids now thought to be diabetic or pre-diabetic the odds aren't in your kiddos favor.

> It's easier to fool people than to convince
> them that they have been fooled.
> – Mark Twain

Whether you see it, or even recognize it, sugar is in just about every product on the supermarket shelf. From bacon to milk, from bread to salad dressing, no really, it's true.

But you can't rely on the food manufacturers to call it sugar. nope, instead, they call it barley malt, dextrose, maltose, sucrose, high-fructose corn syrup, and rice syrup—to name just a few. According to sugarscience.org, sugar comes in at least sixty-one different names! I know, right? Who the heck is running the food industry, Montgomery Burns?

THE CRUELEST CON OF ALL

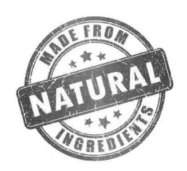

Run from any food whose label boasts "All Natural" for this is the cruelest con of all. It preys on the very people that are trying to make better choices. Sadly, neither the FDA nor the USDA seems keen to police these "all-natural" labels.

As a result, food manufacturers are free to slap a "natural" label on foods that could potentially contain any number of processed ingredients. It may help to think of it this way: 100 years ago, 80% of the food found on supermarket shelves didn't even exist.

Still not convinced, huh?

Unless you have spent the past few years living in a creepy apartment with the curtains closed, you might have also noticed the rest of the outside world is experiencing a surge in food allergies. Maybe it's not food that is the problem, but what's been done to the food that's the problem.

If the bugs won't go near it with a 12ft pole, why are we rushing to fill our carts with it? What is it that the bugs know that we don't? Let's take a closer look.

GMO

The food industry is quick to tell us that GMO crops are safe. While this might even be true, this technology is still in its infancy. As yet, nobody has conducted any long-term studies to back that bold statement up.

As it stands, what we do know is that companies have begun splicing animal bacteria and viral genes with our raw vegetables and fruit. This is something that has never been done before in our history. I know, right? Man messing with our food, what could possibly go wrong?

It's fair to say a good quote will stand the test of time. Who hasn't heard the now famous quote, "Let food be thy medicine and medicine be thy food."? If we are still quoting Hippocrates almost 2500 years later, maybe he knew a thing or two after all. Hippocrates did not say, "Spray thy food with chemicals and then splice it with the bacteria of an animal." Surely that would be utter nonsense.

As you walk the supermarket food aisle, keep in mind that the average vegetable now travels approximately 1500 miles to get to your dinner plate. Then compare it to the food found at your local farmer's market.

To our ancestors, sending food on a 1500 miles trip would have seemed like wasteful folly. Our ancestors understood the value of eating real food and not what today we perceive as food. Keep in mind the Roman army marched on its stomach, not Captain Crunchy.

STALK A SENIOR

Slowly we are moving toward exploring the idea that there are foods that heal and foods that absolutely don't. How do we find the foods that heal? One way to find a diet that works for you is to keep reading my blogs. Another is to find a senior over the age of sixty who still looks healthy.

Think about it, the body can't take six decades of eating junk food and still work and look good. Young people can get away with it and still look good on the outside. Or as Bernard Shaw once said, "Youth is wasted on the young." I digress.

Typically, anyone who's over 60 that is still active has to be doing something right, am I right? If you approach people in the right way, most will be glad to share what it is that keeps them healthy. Be respectful and some seniors may even be flattered that you've even noticed.

Maybe the next time you are standing in line at the supermarket, be on the lookout for anyone who's over sixty and still looks to have radiant health. Don't be stalking now, just smile and take a discreet glance at the things they are buying. Don't be surprised to see a lack of processed foods in their shopping carts.

The most heavily processed foods are pre-made meals—obviously, these include things like frozen pizza and microwaveable dinners. Microwave meals are cheap and quick to make, but cheap food is an illusion if it makes you ill over time.

Astonishingly enough, there is a strong connection between whatever we put into the shopping cart and what ends up in our mouths. Making poor choices in the supermarket all but guarantees that poor choices will be made in the kitchen.

PLEASE DON'T PROD

Now, back in the supermarket line, do you also see that other person, yup, you know the one I'm talking about. The guy whose kids are bouncing off the walls high on sugar. And how does his cart look?

If discretion is a new tool to you, please refrain from pointing or, God forbid, giving in to the urge to start prodding with your organic cucumber. The struggle is real, it happens.

What did we learn from this?
The perception of what is healthy can dramatically vary from one person to another.

Supermarkets are designed to conspire against our subconscious and have become masters of distraction. Sugar is now routinely added to lots of foods, but it's not always called sugar.

Homework: to see what a healthy 60+ man looks like with no shirt on check out a blog by the name of "Mark's Daily Apple" or click on this link. http://www.marksdailyapple.com/

Chapter 18

MEET YOUR TOXIC FUNGI

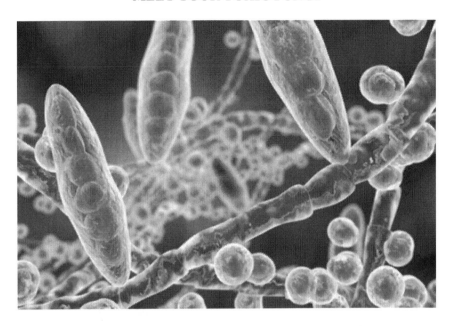

Fungi are persistent and adaptable; effective in all that they do. They can mimic parts of your body and even send out confusing signals to evade detection. Fungi is the plural of fungus and they take on many forms. Whether you realize it or not, dangerous fungi are already living deep inside you.

Infections can spread quickly or slowly, they can be acute or chronic and **some may even turn deadly!**

While there are lots of types of fungi we can break them down into two groups of either superficial or systemic infections. Superficial fungal infections are far more annoying than problematic as they grow on the *outside* of the body. This would affect the nails and surface of the skin.

THE DANGER WITHIN

Systemic infections are more of a concern due to their insidious yet subtle nature. A systemic infection often avoids detection by taking weeks or months to become an issue. Problems often start in the lungs, but in severe cases may spread to the blood, heart, brain, kidneys, and liver. Some reports even suggest that there is a strong a connection between fungus and cancer. Nobel peace prize winner Otto Warburg believed that fungus was *not* a cancer, but it certainly acted like one.

Attempting to eradicate fungi from the body shows a lack of understanding for this formidable foe. Fungi have been a part of this world since the beginning of time. To be clear, there is no ridding yourself of fungi. It might be more prudent to ask, "How is my body going to effectively manage this problem?

In a healthy, well-balanced body, fungi will coexist with little disruption to the host, but fungi are an opportunistic organism. The moment they sense a stressed, malnourished body it will result in a fungal imbalance somewhere. Hear me now, getting the genie back in the bottle is no easy process.

Fungal infections can pop up just about anywhere but tend to occur mostly in moist areas, such as between the toes, in the crotch, or in the mouth. Ever noticed that thick white coating on the tongue? Yup, it's a form of fungi.

Fortunately, the body wants to maintain a state of equilibrium. It works hard to keep fungi in-check by essentially crowding them out with good bacteria. It's a case of having more good guys in your system than bad guys. So long as the balanced doesn't tip in the favor of the fungi life is good.

Like so many battles, this isn't one you can win, it has to be controlled. At this point, you should be asking yourself, what the heck would tip the balance in their favor?

That a great question and the answer is twofold. The first is fungi thrives on sugar. An obvious smart first step in the right direction is to limit their preferred food supply. Here's where it gets tricky.

Sugar is now systematically hidden in everyday food items. It can be found in frozen yogurt, baked beans, bread, soup, salad dressing, sushi, even some brands of bacon! Are you catching all this? Sugar *isn't* just cookies, candy, and soda!

But sugar *isn't* the problem per se, it's the amount of sugar that causes the problem. When the amount of sugar overshadows the body's ability to regulate it, the balance is tipped. Given that the average soda drink contains the equivalent of seven teaspoons of sugar, tipping the balance isn't that difficult to do.

Let's not forget that even "healthy" fruit juices are nothing more than liquid sugar. To add to the problem, all carbohydrates turn to sugar and even protein turns to sugar. *No really, it's true.*

TO THE BATTLEGROUND

For now, let's go back to those fungi—you know, the ones already living inside you. Think of them as small groups of dangerous rebels who like to feed on sugar. In a healthy body they are surrounded by an army of good bacteria and so the threat remains pretty low.

But, those rebel fungi always have aspirations to overthrow the government (that's you.) This battle plays out daily in the gut. So long as fungi remain vastly outnumbered by the good guys, the body can keep them at a manageable level.

But fungi have learned how to wait. Once the right opportunity presents itself, fungi will spring into action and develop a stronghold. As their numbers begin to swell, the trail of destruction has the potential to tear down the whole system (yup, unfortunately, you again).

THIS WILL ACT AS A SPRINGBOARD FOR FUNGI

Keeping fungi in check is a challenge at the best of times—when we add the second part to this problem all bets are off. Statistically speaking, you have probably already made this mistake. *Any guesses what it is?*

Hands up anyone who's ever taken antibiotics for a viral infection. Don't get me wrong, when used correctly, antibiotics can help save lives. But they are sometimes handed out for the wrong reason. In case you missed the memo, antibiotics are useless at fighting viruses. Antibiotics are good at fighting bad bacteria but they also kill indiscriminately (that's not so good).

When antibiotics become over prescribed it can help fungi get a firm foothold. With each prescription for antibiotics, it may even create super-strength bacteria (and in some cases, it already has). This new super-bacteria, will, in turn, become resistant to all forms of antibiotics. **But there's another problem, can you see it?**

Even if you choose not to take antibiotics, the problem isn't entirely eliminated. How so?

Antibiotics are now heavily used in the food supply (oh come on) and if the animals we eat consume antibiotics, then so do we. This type of antibiotic overuse has the potential to solve one problem but create another.

To be clear, antibiotic overuse is a recipe for disaster. Once we decide to disproportionately kill off large groups of gut bacteria, our health will suffer. Here's another way to look at the problem. The word "anti" means against, biotic pertains to life, in this context we could think of antibiotics as being anti-life.

A constant craving for sugar may be an indicator that an imbalance has already begun. Pathogenic bacteria, parasites, and yeast, such as candida feed off sugar. The more sugar you eat, the more inviting you make your gut for these "bad guys."

The good news is, when you learn to pay attention, fungus becomes an excellent teacher. Usually, a body with a superficial fungal infection will itch, almost to the point where you could scratch through the skin whenever sugar is consumed. Are you getting this? Your body is so smart it's telling you when you get it wrong.

PROBIOTICS

While it's unfortunate that antibiotics wreak havoc on our delicate ecosystem it may be possible to readjust the balance in the favor of the good guys. Hoorah!

Good guys are aided when we consume fermented foods but it does take time. Probiotics may help speed things up a little by helping to repopulate the good bacteria. As with most things, you get what you pay for, so don't be too surprised if that "bargain" brand probiotic at the box store doesn't do it for you. The better probiotics are often found in health food stores.

It's better to buy the best probiotics you can afford rather than what's on sale. This is your health and as such, it needs to have a value. Some probiotics can be heat or moisture sensitive, and some may need refrigeration. With that in mind, it's a good idea not to leave probiotics sitting in your hot car or out on the kitchen counter.

MASTERS OF SURVIVAL

There are lots of different fungus types but all are masters of survival. If they have one quality above all others it is this: they know how to adapt. Put simply, yeast cells aren't going to just roll over and die for you while your sugar levels are elevated.
The fungus you may have heard most about is candida—and it's already living inside you. But candida can easily get out of control, when this happens, watch out!

Candida comes in the form of yeast (a microscopic fungus) that lives in the intestines. When it's kept in check its primary function is to assist with digestion and the absorption of nutrients. It coexists with good

181

bacteria and, all things being equal, the two live happily together. But it's a delicate balance and problems start when candida gets a little too big for its boots.

When presented with the right opportunity, candida will quickly become invasive. As soon as it has the upper hand, a cascade of problems follows. Out of control candida breaks down the wall of the intestine, it releases toxic byproducts into your bloodstream. Well, hello again to you, cheeky-leaky gut.

A diet that's high in carbohydrates will favor candida, as will sustained levels of stress, antibiotics, alcohol consumption, and oral contraceptives. And hello to you, Mr. Estrogen disruptor.

CANDIDA

To make a candida outbreak all the more interesting, taking fermented foods won't help. In fact, this time around, they may even make things worse. This is due in part to an increased Herxheimer reaction, sometimes called a "die-off" reaction.

When a die-off occurs, metabolic by-products are released into the body. When the candida yeast cells die, they release 79 different toxins, including ethanol and acetaldehyde.

It might surprise you to know that the health drink kombucha, favored by many health freaks, can add to the problem. *Why?*
Kombucha contains wild strains of yeast and, due to the activity of the yeast, is also slightly alcoholic. The immune system of someone struggling with Candida overgrowth may find it a challenge to deal with these wild strains of yeast.

Die-off symptoms can include the following.

- Nausea
- Headache, fatigue, dizziness
- Swollen glands
- Bloating, gas, constipation, or diarrhea

- Increased joint or muscle pain
- Elevated heart rate
- Chills, cold feeling in your extremities
- Body itchiness, hives, or rashes
- Sweating
- Fever
- Skin breakouts
- Recurring vaginal, prostate, and sinus infections

A candida diet will prove helpful. But the moment die-off symptoms begin is the time when most people prematurely abandon their candida diet.

Low energy and brain fog are classic symptoms of a candida overgrowth. Usually accompanied with strong cravings for cookies, candy, and bread. AKA sugar. Sugar has an addictive quality to it much the same as any ugly street drug.

GOOD NEWS TEST

The good news is; I have a clear way to test yourself for candida. You can even do it in the comfort of your own home without it costing you a dime. Ready?

Before going to bed fill a clear glass with water, allow it to stand overnight at room temperature. Next, pin a note to your bathroom mirror to remind you to spit into the glass first thing in the morning. Do this BEFORE you eat, drink, or brush your teeth.

The trick is to accumulate enough saliva in your mouth and then with the glass held close to your mouth gently spit the saliva into the glass of water. I know right, gross, but watch carefully, the sample saliva is then going to do one of three things.

(1) Float on the top of the water
(2) Sink to the bottom
(3) Slowly make its way downward and begin looking like it's growing jellyfish type legs

So far so good, now give it five minutes and then hold the glass up to the daylight from the bathroom window. This will help you see the result more clearly. If the spit remains floating on the top, then the spit test suggests you are free of candida.

If it's sinking or growing jellyfish-type legs, it suggests a candida presence. To ensure accuracy, this test should be carried out for six consecutive mornings.

If candida is confirmed, you could also ask your doctor to check for you for candida. This is done by running a blood test to check your levels of antibodies called IgG, IgA, and IgM. At this point DON'T get too freaked out if you test positive, most of us do and it's totally manageable. Remember, cutting out sugar is ALWAYS a smart first step in the right direction.

Treating any type of fungi is a marathon race, not a sprint. It takes time and effort but the rewards for getting this step right are real. If you want to keep fungi in check, then here's the part that you need to contribute to.

For the next six weeks keep your sugar intake to an absolute minimum. Yup, that includes fruit, which is loaded with natural sugars. While we are at it, cut out those other "healthy" sugars such as honey, agave syrup, and even our old friend maple syrup.

The goal is to starve fungi. This will not only benefit your gut but also your immune system, thyroid, and adrenal glands. Once you have the amount of sugar reduced, treating candida with specific probiotics may also prove helpful. To do this correctly, be sure to invest in a quality brand that contains a strain of Saccharomyces Boulardii.

Often it is labeled simply as S Boulardii. Saccharomyces Boulardii (to use its full name). It's a friendly yeast that binds to the same sites on the intestinal wall lining as candida does, effectively crowding it out. S. Boulardii has also been shown to be helpful in the treatment of diarrhea, IBS, and IBD.

184

The key here is to do things gradually by slowly building up the dose of S. Boulardii. This will help keep any unpleasant symptoms of die-off to a minimum.

As always, start with a small dose and go slow. By this I mean don't take a mega dose, and whenever you take any form of probiotic supplements, be sure to space out the times.

Candida can also be fought with the help of food grade diatomaceous earth and bentonite red clay. Both of these will prove themselves to be useful allies and are discussed in more detail later. Typically, I'm not a fan of using too many things at the same time, simply because it can cause the body to go out of balance.

As with any new supplement, some people will do better than others, which is why I'll always give you several options to try. When used sensibly, GSE (grape seed extract) is another powerful anti-fungal tool. It can sometimes be helpful in killing sugar cravings.

Whenever problems in the gut are addressed, it might also be a good idea to stay close to the bathroom, especially if you have a sensitive system. This should work itself out and the bigger picture
It is estimated that 70% of us live with a candida overgrowth and contrary to popular belief it affects both men and women. Some of the typical symptoms are:

- Strong cravings for sugar and refined carbohydrates
- Frequent brain fog and inability to concentrate
- Digestive issues such as bloating, constipation, or diarrhea
- Feeling tired and worn out all the time
- A white coat on tongue
- Difficulty concentrating, poor memory, lack of focus, ADD, ADHD
- Skin issues like eczema, psoriasis, hives, and rashes
- Irritability, mood swings
- Anxiety or depression
- Severe seasonal allergies or itchy ears
- Fibromyalgia
- Athlete's foot or toenail fungus

- Bad breath
- Hormone imbalance
- Joint pain
- Loss of sex drive
- Chronic sinus and allergy issues
- Urinary tract infections, rectal itching, or vaginal itching
- Weakened immune system
- Autoimmune diseases such as Hashimoto's thyroiditis, rheumatoid arthritis, ulcerative colitis, lupus, psoriasis, or multiple sclerosis

Phew, that's quite a list! That white coating on the tongue is a particular giveaway that something funky is going, on or that something is out of balance.

What did we learn from this?
Fungi come in many different forms. It takes a sustained effort to rid the body of the worst of them, but once fungi are in check, good health will flourish.

Cutting out sugar and restricting antibiotic use is a great start in the fight against fungi.
In order for the body to deal with fungi, it needs to be in balance. Too much or too little of anything can be a bad thing. This is something we will continue to explore in more detail.

Homework: Check out Christa Orecchio for an effective candida protocol. https://www.youtube.com/watch?v=HjymtezoWH8

Chapter 19

WHATS EATING YOU ALIVE?

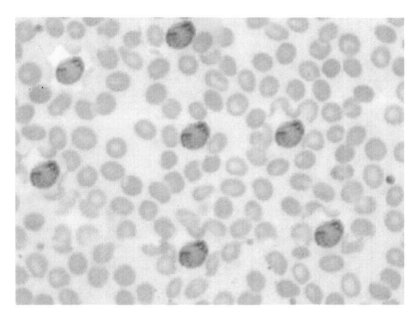

As we learned in the last chapter, fungi can have far-reaching detrimental effects on our health. But fungi have a bunch of toxic cousins and I just know you won't like the sound of them.

Parasites come in all shapes and sizes; some microscopic and you wouldn't even know if you had them. The largest can grow up to 82 feet (25m) long. Thankfully, anything that size is quite rare. But the smaller ones?

Meh, not so rare.

How many different types of parasites are there? - Science is still counting, some estimates suggest it can run into the thousands, if not tens of thousands. The only thing we do know for sure is that they can affect everyone from adorable babies to reliable old grandpa's.

If you have ever swum in a stream, kept a dog, or been on holiday abroad your risk actually increases. This can create something of a disconnect when trying to find the source of a parasitic infection. Let's not forget that we could also be looking for something the size of a pinhead!

Still not convinced, huh?

Check this out. Two decades ago in the U.S. a parasite entered Milwaukee drinking water and killed 69 people and sickened 400,000. More recently, in 2015, a potentially deadly amoeba was found in the water supply of a parish outside New Orleans (for the second time in two years). This is real folks, and it can happen in any town or city across the globe.

The deadliest parasite known to man is airborne. The World Health Organization (WHO), estimates that malaria killed 438,000 people in 2015 alone. Yup, malaria is spread by a parasite. No really, it's true.

We like to think of parasites as a third world problem, but today the world has become a much smaller place. Food is flown and shipped around the world with ease and parasites travel visa free. This opens the door to parasites from the food you eat and the water you drink.

Undercooked pork is particularly susceptible. To be sure, commercial pig farming is a barbaric practice at the best of times. Ironically, filthy inhumane living conditions are not how the pig would choose to live. My point is this, be careful where you buy your meat from. Local pasture raised meat is better by a country mile.
What's the biggest cause of a parasitic infection? - An underperforming immune system.

GOOD NEWS

Fortunately, a parasite and worm cleanse is easy enough to do. Effective cleanses can be found in your local health food store. You can also seek the services of a healthcare professional. If for any reason that path takes you on a fruitless mission, you could also look into "Zapping".

This is a small battery operated device but unlike the name suggests, it's quite harmless to you. To parasites, not so much. It works by emitting a very low range frequency onto the skin which is thought to disrupts parasite cycles.

A basic zapping unit starts around $50. A top of the line zapper can get unnecessarily expensive. You can find out more about parasite zappers with a simple google search. Combining the zapper with a parasite cleanse may prove more effective.

DIATOMACEOUS EARTH

If your budget is running a little tight be sure to check out food grade diatomaceous earth. As an added bonus, it brings to the table other health benefits. Diatomaceous earth may also prove helpful fungi as well as parasites making it a win/win.

It's imperative that you buy only FOOD GRADE diatomaceous earth. It's actually as cheap as chips. A one-pound bag sells for around 10 bucks. Diatomaceous earth is best taken on an empty stomach in the morning with water. The dose may vary depending on your size, age and weight so always consult the company you buy it from.

Diatomaceous earth is a white, porous, sedimentary rock, naturally-made from the fossilized remains of diatoms. Diatomaceous earth may also help with bowel movements; some people say they "just feel better" after consuming it. That said, best results are often experienced when by rotating consumption, ten days on, ten days off.

Depending on how congested you are, it may take a week or so before you begin to see more regular bowel movements. When done correctly, an effective parasite protocol lifts the burden off the immune system and may even help curb those junk food cravings.

What did we learn from this?
Parasites are a part of our world. They can steal vital nutrients and kill millions of people.

Homework: watch a short Discovery documentary called "Parasites Eating Us Alive" Paperback homies you can find this on YouTube. https://www.youtube.com/watch?v=w_D6yPVrYjo

Chapter 20

UNDERSTANDING FOOD

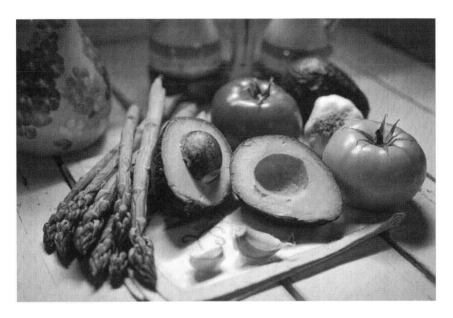

Before we rush into talking about the *any* diet in any detail, we first need to have a clear understanding of food groups. On the surface groups such as carbohydrates, fats, fiber, and even protein may all seem pretty straightforward. But scratch below the surface and these terms are often misunderstood or used in the wrong context.

Our first example is "fruitsandvegetables." This isn't a typo; it's written that way because people often refer to them as if they were the same thing. Fruit gets people into trouble because of its high sugar content, even more so when it's been dried out. For anyone looking to follow the ketogenic diet, it may help to think fruit as a watery bags of sugar. That "organic" fruit juice doesn't fare much better which is essentially a form of liquid sugar.

In most western diets, fruits are typically over-consumed and vegetables are under-consumed. This wasn't how our ancestors ate, back then, eating fruit out of season, would have seen you stoned as a witch, and rightly so.

Today we think nothing of picking up a carton of ripe strawberries in the dead of winter. Which loops back nicely to people eating too much fruit. To be clear, fruit can spike your sugar and kick you out of ketosis faster than a speeding ticket. Yes, berries are lower on the glycemic table, but it doesn't take too many to put you back on the sugar train. Chew-chew (sorry, bad joke).

VEGETABLES

When choosing vegetables pay particular attention to their bold colors. As a rule of thumb, any vegetable that has the same color running all the way through it has a higher nutrient density. No really, it's true.

It's often said that variety is the spice of life, it's also pretty good for the gut biome. A nice expression to remember is to try and "eat the rainbow." Think of red carrots on a plate next to slices of beets with vibrant green green lettuce, red onion, and yellow peppers (if you can handle them). As a side note, some may find that too many raw veggies irritate the gut lining, if this is you, lightly cook or stream them. That said, certain "leafy greens" are best uncooked as they can help the body to detoxify.

FATS AND OILS

The ketogenic diet is all about the fat. But there is more to this important nutrient than meets the eye. Straight out of the gate, it's important to note that not all fats are the same; there are good fats and there are bad fats.

The word "fat" is often used as a blanket term that does a great disservice to this important nutrient. Over the years, fat has been demonized, I'm sure we have all seen those "low fat" labels in the supermarket.

But clearly we need good fat because important vitamins like A, E, D and K are all fat-soluble — simply put, good fats help us absorb those important vitamins. Perhaps this is why Mother Nature hides so much fat in breast milk. Hmm, I see.

Just to keep things interesting, fats can also be split into two more groups containing saturated fat and unsaturated fat. Rather than allowing this to get complicated let's stick with using the term's good and bad. What we don't need are those manmade fats such as trans-fats or partially hydrogenated vegetable oils. These are "bad-fats" and can be found in margarine and vegetable shortening.

Fast food restaurants also like to cook with them because they are cheap. But the body really can't handle these types of fats and they quickly begin to mess with our chemistry. For any foggy thinkers out there, know that your brain is made up of approximately 60% fat. Trust me, stay away from bad fats. Those mother-fatters will mess with your mind.

Brains do much better with good fats, hence the ketogenic diet is loaded with them. People are often surprised to learn that the standard ketogenic diet or SKD for short, typically contains 75% (good) fat, 20% protein and only 5% carbs.

One of the most common mistakes keto newbies tend to make is thinking that low carb means eating more meat. As you can see from the ratio above, this simply isn't the case. I know what you are thinking because I had the same thought, where the heck do I find 75% of good fat?

It's actually not that difficult. You can pick up lots of good fats by eating certain fish, especially wild caught salmon, (or sardines if you are on a tight budget). Good fat can also be found in raw nuts such as the macadamia nut, and in fatty meats, olives, eggs, and yup, let's not forget avocados. One medium avocado has approximately 23 grams of fat.

If you find yourself in a bind, more fat can come in the form of coconut cream. It's sold in a can and has 14g of good fat. Obviously, we want a brand that has no added sugar.

With a little imagination (along with a bit of time in the freezer), coconut cream can almost taste like ice cream. Throw in a handful of nuts (or a few berries from the lower end of the glycemic table) and you have just made a treat that keeps hunger at bay.

Another great source of good fat is a concentrated version of coconut oil, often called MCT oil (Medium-Chain-Triglycerides). MCT oil may also prove helpful with mental clarity. Some folks add it their salad, others add a tablespoon into their coffee. As with anything new, start small and go slow.

For this next good fat, I'm going to break with the standard mantra and also call butter a beneficial fat. I'll explain the logic of this in a later. The good news is if you are lactose intolerant you may find that butter from pasture-fed cows (such as Kerrygold) is better tolerated.

Cheese is yet another good fat, but those with sensitivities should still avoid it (even if it is pasture raised). If this is you, be sure to check out goat's cheese which some people seem to fair much better with.

More good fat comes in the form of omega-3 fatty acids, which our bodies cannot produce. The two crucial ones are EPA and DHA, these are well-known for their anti-inflammatory benefits. If you are trying to limit the number of fish products in your diet because you have concerns about heavy metal toxicity, a good source of essential DHA and EPA omega-3 fatty acids is krill oil. Generally speaking, krill oil is lower in contaminants.

Omega-3s can also be found in chia seeds, flax seeds, and walnuts. Pasture-raised eggs have been shown to contain more Omega-3 fatty acids and vitamin-A than regular factory farmed eggs.

This early on I don't want us to get sucked down an omega-3 rabbit hole as we still have so much to cover. But it's good to know that a healthy balance of omega-3 and omega-6 is something that needs to be addressed. An incorrect balance may increase inflammation in the body. As a rule of thumb, strive for a balance of 1:1 which is better than an excessive imbalance. Good luck getting there, if you follow the standard American diet (SAD) as it has waaaay too many omega-6s and not enough omega-3s. Some estimates put the imbalance as far out as 40:1 in favor of omega-6s. Ahhh, ignorance is bliss, until it kills you!

In the past, people were all a little quick to follow a low-fat diet. Some nutrition experts suggest that the current food pyramid would actually be more beneficial if it were turned upside down. Make no mistake, good fat is important to your health.

Eating more good fat also helps us feel fuller longer. It slows down the absorption of carbohydrates which in turn helps keep blood sugar levels under control. For that reason, diabetics may also do well with the ketogenic diet.

Before we move onto the next food group, I just want to add that the correct way to increase good fat in your diet is by doing it gradually. As with anything new, always start small and go slow (I'll continue using this term like a broken record because it's super important). Ultimately, we all have different needs and, for some, consuming too much good fat when the body isn't used to it can present a new problem — a stressed gallbladder. A good clue for this is usually a pain in the right shoulder. I digress.

PROTEIN

Protein is protein, right? *Meh, not so fast.*

Often times the word "protein" is inaccurately used to describe meat, and even then is applied with an enormously liberal brush. Technically speaking, protein can be found in spider venom, yuk, who wants to put that in a crock-pot?

Also, deep fried chicken can be called a protein. But let's not forget that it's usually fried in rancid oils (bad fat) which can be an instant hit of inflammation-forming free radicals.

Let's take protein a step further.

Humans and gorillas are genetically very similar; we actually share 98% of our genes with them. An adult silverback gorilla can weigh 500+ pounds and is estimated to be twenty times stronger than an adult man, yet gorillas don't eat chickens or cows. And yet, gorillas are composed mostly of muscle with a fat content of just 3%.

So where does their muscle building protein comes from? Well, it's not KFC that's for sure. It comes from the sixteen pounds of plants and leaves they eat every single day. Yup, protein can absolutely be found in vegetation. I know, right? Who knew?

Am I saying we should all become a vegetarian? Nope, never did say that. However, the perception that any diet consisting of vegetables is somehow inferior needs to be challenged. Think about it, the muscle that powers a racehorse is also formed without consuming any meat. As any vegan bodybuilder will tell you, meat is not the only way to get protein.

Again, I'm not attempting to convert meat eaters into vegetarians or vegetarians into meat eaters. I'm simply challenging your perception of what protein is.

Bottom line: yes, protein can be found in meat, but not all meats are the same. Keep this in mind as we move through the rest of these food groups. There is always going to be a junk version and a healthy version.

Pasture-raised meat is a term used to describe the way an animal has been raised. It simply means it's been left to graze as nature intended. When it comes to buying meat, try to support local farmers who allow their animals to be raised on open pastures. If you can't afford the sticker price of a farmer doing his job right, then the solution is to eat less meat. That's okay too, but don't forget, when the animal you eat consumes antibiotics, so do you.

Tip 1 — Always keep meat on the bottom shelf of your fridge, that way if it leaks for any reason it's not going to drip on your vegetables and make you sick.

Tip 2— If meat doesn't smell right to you, get rid of it. Remember the golden rule. If in doubt, throw it out.

FIBER and STARCH

Even though both starch and fiber are complex carbs, they act very differently in your body. If you are looking for something to give you energy, starchy food may help. If you want something filling that isn't loaded with calories, opt for something high in fiber.

Here's why.

Enzymes in your body can easily break the bonds that form starches, turning them into sugars for energy. But your body can't make enzymes to break down fiber, so fiber isn't fully digested — but it does have some health benefits. This would include lowering your risk for heart disease, high blood pressure, and obesity.

FIBER

Fiber is important, not least to aid in good digestion. Unfortunately, much of the standard dietary advice often lists breakfast cereal and whole grain bread as good forms of fiber. While it may be true that the fiber content in these foods is high, so too is the possibility of a reaction, particularly from gluten. Don't panic, I'll cover food triggers soon enough.

There are lots of alternative sources of fiber. Quinoa is gluten-free, high in fiber, and has a higher nutrient content than most grains. Oatmeal made from gluten-free oats also has fiber, but be aware that many of the "instant" brands can be loaded with additives and sugar. While standard oats may take a few minutes longer to prepare, they are generally better tolerated. Soaking oats overnight can help turn them into instant oats. In the morning simply strain out the water and replace with warm almond milk.

As a rule of thumb, oatmeal will bump you out of ketosis but that in itself isn't always a bad thing. Some folks tend to cycle their carbs which means they go full ketogenic followed by a few days of slightly higher carbs. This is also known as the cyclical ketogenic diet (CKD): typically, this is five days keto two days with higher carbs. For me personally, I try to listen to my own body, I kinda get a feel for when I need to carb up and when to stretch it out.

The value of fiber shouldn't be underestimated because it helps to support your gut microbiome. This is a complex ecosystem of bacteria located within our bodies. The vast majority of the bacterial species live in our digestive system. This is a super interesting area of medicine and perhaps one day I'll write another book on this very topic. But for now, let's not bite off more than we can chew (intended pun).

Fiber can also be found in plant foods like vegetables, cooked turnip greens, spinach, beans, chickpeas, lentils, and nuts. For those who can tolerate it, brown rice has more fiber than white rice. If you struggle with bloating from rice it may be helpful to buy "sprouted rice." There's a pretty good one sold here in the US called "Sprouted Blonde Gaba Rice" from Planet Rice. I have zero affiliation with this company so feel free to check out other sprouted rice. As always, I'm just trying to save you a little time.

Fiber can also be found in fruits such as avocado, pears, apples, blueberries, and raspberries.

STARCH

Starches are a complex carbohydrate (I'll get to those in a moment), so let's keep this one short and simple. Vegetables high in starches are also generally higher in calories. Starches are found in vegetables such as potatoes, broccoli, Brussels sprouts, peas, parsnips, green beans, dried beans, and corn. Side note, some estimates also suggest that 90% of corn is now genetically modified. For some folks, corn is notoriously harsh on the digestive system. Hmm, I see.

SIMPLE AND COMPLEX CARBOHYDRATES

Simply put, we could think of carbs as one or more sugar molecules bound together and then broken down by the body to be used as fuel. ALL carbs turn to sugar, some faster than others.

Carbohydrates (or carbs for short) are found in lots of different foods. They are in fruits, grains, vegetables, pastries, potatoes, bread, and even milk, candy, and soda. Carbs can then be split into two basic groups, either simple or complex. Shall we take a look?

Simple carbs are easily absorbed into the bloodstream because of their simple molecular structure. Think fruit, milk, table sugar, etc. Simple carbs can be thought of as giving you a faster hit of sugar.

Complex carbs have a more complex molecular structure that can take longer for the body to break down into sugar. Think grains, vegetables, potatoes, etc. Complex carbs can be thought of as giving you a slower hit of sugar. So far we have simple carbs and complex carbs, now we need to split them once again into good carbs and bad carbs. I know right, but this bit is super easy.

In the interest of simplicity, let us think of bad carbs as those that have been heavily processed. This would include cereals, crackers, pastries, white bread, soda, etc. Bad carbs are high in calories but essentially low in nutrients.

This now gets easier because it only leaves good carbs. Good carbs are the unprocessed foods such as fruits, vegetables, beans, etc., and are always found in their natural state.

SUGAR AND SPICE

SUGAR is a tricky one because as we learned earlier it can be just as addictive as cocaine! Food manufacturers know this, which is perhaps why sugar is added to everyday items like milk, bacon, bread, and even salad dressing. To make matters worse, you can't even rely on sugar to be called sugar by the people whose job it is to write the labels.

Here are a few of the common bait and switch terms used for sugar —
but there are plenty more! Cane Juice, Corn sweetener, Corn syrup,
Dextrose, Fructose, High-fructose corn syrup, Invert sugar, Maltose,
Lactose, Sucrose, White sugar, Corn syrup solids, malt syrup, Anhydrous
dextrose, yadda, yadda, yadda.

If you aren't paying attention, all this sugar quickly adds up to a body
that can no longer cope. The medical term for that is diabetes.
Remember, carbs (and to a lesser degree protein) are also broken down
into sugar.

You can find a FULL list of the sugar content of foods in the glycemic
index table. The glycemic index table is a value assigned to foods based
on how slowly or how quickly those foods cause increases in blood
glucose levels. Also known as "blood sugar" levels.

SPICE

Turmeric is arguably one of the most studied and powerful spices on the
planet. Turmeric has been used in cooking for thousands of years. It has
a warm, peppery, and bitter flavor and a mild fragrance slightly
reminiscent of orange and ginger. The main active ingredient in turmeric
is cucumin which has powerful anti-inflammatory effects and is a very
strong antioxidant. Turmeric is fat-soluble which means you want to take
it with food that has a certain level of fat content. This will allow the
turmeric to better absorbed. Turmeric/curcumin has long been studied for
its cancer preventative properties. Adding turmeric to your food is easy
to do and is thought to have wide-ranging beneficial effects. However,
quality is key. **Many herbs and spices coming from India and China
are known to contain alarming amounts of lead!** Keep in mind that the
organic label is no guarantee that a product is free of heavy metals, it
simply suggests its free of pesticides

There are lots of herbs and spices with health benefits, enough to warrant
a whole chapter on the subject. Given that we still have a lot to cover I'll
just surface brush a couple of them.

Other useful spices known to have health benefits are cinnamon, ginseng, and ginger. Ginger has an astounding number of health benefits. It can aid digestion and speed up metabolism. It's also antibacterial, ant parasitic. Garlic is also another well researched antibacterial and anti-parasitic. Due to the high sulfur content in garlic, it can be helpful with detoxification. That said, garlic is also a potent lectin which can be a problem for some individuals.

FISH

Try to limit your fish consumption to those kinds that are known to be lower in mercury. Wild caught salmon from Alaska is a good choice, although any fish with a high selenium content can be consumed in moderation.

Selenium plays a role in counteracting mercury toxicity, something we have known about for more than forty-five years. Sardines fall in the high selenium category, but avoid fish such as swordfish, shark, king mackerel, and tilefish. To be on the safe side, limit tuna to once every two weeks or less.

NUTS AND SEEDS

Be mindful not to consume too many nuts in one sitting. Doing so will almost certainly throw your balance of omega-3 and omega-6 fats into a bad ratio. Anthropological research suggests that our hunter-gatherer ancestors consumed omega-6 and omega-3 fats in a ratio of roughly 1.1.

When it comes to eating nuts, moderation may serve you better than excess. Think how long it would have taken our ancestors to crack open a single nut. Today it's possible to consume large amounts of nuts because all the hard work of removing the shell has been done for us. Keep in mind that peanuts and pistachios are both prone to mold.

Sprouted seeds are less problematic than un-sprouted seeds. If you are looking for an economical way to bring an abundance of minerals and live enzymes into your diet.

FERMENTED FOODS

Fermented foods are packed with good probiotics and can help boost the number of good bacteria found in your gut. Fermented foods also have the ability to positively influence the immune system, but it's better to gradually work your way up. As in the case of candida, too many fermented foods too quickly could hasten a die-off reaction.

Some estimates put the weight of the tiny gut microorganisms at approximately three pounds per person! Given the extraordinary ability of the gut to affect both our physical and mental health, any attempts to influence the gut flora can produce a certain amount of unpredictability. Better to start small and go slow.

CALORIES

Looking at food as a number is too much of a one-dimensional approach to nutrition. Calorie counting fails to take into account the quality of the food because it focuses instead on a measurement of energy.

While it's obviously important to have enough calories coming into the diet, the obsession with calorie counting has the potential to become counterproductive. Stop counting calories and start counting quality!

RICE AND GRAINS

Rice is a borderline trigger food that some people do okay with and in others can prove reactive. If this is you try giving the rice a vacation for thirty days, and then gradually reintroduce it back.

Grains — Nope, no grains. The ones used in today's food simply aren't the same quality they were even thirty years ago. In some remote parts of Europe, you might get away with it, but for the rest of us? Meh, grains have become an ugly form of kryptonite.

VINEGAR

The healing properties of vinegar date back thousands of years and were used by the Egyptians and Greeks; even Hippocrates used it.

Apple cider vinegar is great for helping food taste better, it's also a powerful tonic to keep in the cupboard. Acetate is a molecule found in apple cider vinegar that has been shown to increase metabolism. Acetate is made by good bacteria in the gut and science is just discovering its use in calming down an overactive immune system.

Many of these claims are backed up with legitimate scientific studies and data can be found on sites such as PubMed. From asthma to migraines (and a whole lot of stuff in between), some people report remarkable improvements from using this type of vinegar.

Apple cider vinegar (sometimes called ACV) can also be helpful for detoxing the body and fighting infection. It's also believed that apple cider vinegar helps the process of digestion become more effective.

Personally, I've found ACV helpful with seasonal allergies. I simply added a tablespoon in a small (16oz) BPA-free bottle of water and kept sipping on it until I found relief. To some, I'm sure it's not going to taste that great, but if you catch allergies early in the season it can be better than itching eyes and sneezing.

Some people report improvement in arthritis, high cholesterol, and even regulating blood pressure. Apple cider vinegar is best diluted in water and drunk on an empty stomach. A good starting point would be a tablespoon in 8 oz. of water. This will also help the minerals in other foods be better absorbed.

For a complete list of effective ACV, remedies be sure to check out a website by the name of earthclinic.com. I used this site often as it's packed with helpful tips and so easy to navigate.

SALT

Salt is often demonized but salt isn't the problem, very often it's the type of salt that creates the problem. Regular table salt is heavily processed and usually contains numerous additives to prevent clumping. Regular table salt has fewer natural minerals than Himalayan salt. By comparison, Himalayan salt also tastes better.

Before we leave this chapter, I'd like to encourage you to put what you have just learned into practice. The next meal you eat, take a moment to see which food groups are on your plate. When we are just starting out it's not uncommon to find our plate stacked with bad carbs, grains, dairy, or fructose in the form of fruit. I know, right? WTF? (Where's The Fat?)

If this is all new to you then as a basic rule of thumb, try to fill half your plate with leafy green vegetables. This will begin to make you view the remaining on your plate as important nutrients.

What did we learn from this?
Food is divided into different groups and each has the potential to affect the body in one way or another. Remembering that some foods can belong to more than one group.

The important take-home message is that sugar comes to us in many forms, all of which we need to dial down. Good fats, however, are like a long lost friend to be welcomed through the door.

Homework: to help cement what we have just learned, there's a super helpful video on YouTube called "Gut reaction part 1." It is well worth watching because it makes understanding this whole chapter easier.
https://www.youtube.com/watch?v=f3iOlRUQkrw&t=345s

Chapter 21

THE FACE OF ADVERSITY

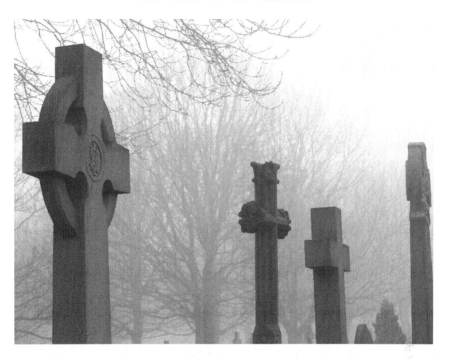

As we now find ourselves at the halfway point in the book, what-say we take a right turn here and see where it takes us. This short chapter shouldn't be at all hard to read because you will not be asked to learn anything new. For now, just take it easy as we ponder this life together.

Getting this book to the point where I'm okay to share it with you took me far longer than I ever expected – a little over a year to be precise. A lot can happen in a year and my dad just died. It's fair to say that the day we buried him I also buried a part of myself. Dad was a genuinely decent man and I'll miss him.

It got me thinking how Dads life had been anything but easy. But to his credit, he rarely complained about anything, he simply wasn't wired that way.

As a teenager, he broke his back and spent six months in a cast. He was lucky to walk again, but as a result of that early injury, he spent the rest of his life in pain. He absolutely point-blank refused to complain about it or even let it stop him from being active. On his 50th birthday, he even began running marathons.

As a way to cope with his pain, he often used humor. Some of his jokes were so bad they were actually quite funny. I once asked him how much it cost to get married and without missing a beat he said, "I'm really not too sure son, I'm still paying for it." He'd been married to my mom for more than sixty years and with some degree of predictability, he always joked that the first fifty-nine were the hardest.

Mom and Dad were inseparable best friends, in all their time together, they never spent a night apart. So the day Dad complained of chest pain they even went off to the doctor together. The doctor shook her head and immediately sent them to the hospital for more testing. Legend has it that they even rode in the ambulance together, holding hands.

Once there, Dad was put through a pretty intense examination. It was then deemed necessary to keep him for observation. Now separated from each other, Dad quickly found himself being prodded and poked by a team of eager medical students. The following morning, I managed to call him while he was still on the ward. When I asked how he was doing, he mentioned that having a large needle plunged into his left lung kinda hurt. Because he so rarely complained, I knew this must have hurt him even more than he was saying.

Dad was then told to drink Barium. If you haven't heard of this before, Barium is used in medicine to highlight any defects during an X-ray. It's also used as an insoluble additive in oil well drilling. It's even added to fireworks to make that bright green color! One of the known side effects of drinking Barium is it can cause a hiatal hernia (an internal defect that causes the stomach to slide partially into the chest).

Despite the risks (and being eighty years old), Dad was asked to drink a second batch. The doctors then carried out yet another round of high radiation x-rays. Once finished, they drew more blood for a standard panel of bloodwork.

The next time I called him he asked me to pray for him, only this time there was no punchline. This struck me as quite odd because neither of us had been inside a church for quite some time. I could only guess that the tests they were now constantly running on him had become pretty intense.

Later that evening I called Dad again.

His mind had always been as sharp as a tack and as we talked I noticed his thoughts were wandering off track. As the conversation unfolded it became clear that he had been given heavy-duty painkillers. After the liquid Barium sulfate, I began to wonder how his liver and kidneys would cope.

A week later Dad had been seen by six specialists. When all his test results were in, all six sat around him in a semi-circle and each told him he was going to die.

Dad had always been a very positive man and rarely expressed any outward sign of emotion that might cause others around him to worry. My sister told me that as he heard the doctors' news, his large square shoulders suddenly dropped. His heart was still beating but I believe this was the exact moment that he lost all hope. Following that damning diagnosis, his beautiful, determined inner spirit begun to wither. He was then sent home.

As if he hadn't been through enough already, a day nurse then came to visit him at the house. She brought with her a signed order to inject him twice a day with warfarin. This was deemed necessary to prevent blood clots. My suggestion that Hawthorne would be a better fit for an eighty-year-old was immediately scoffed at.

Emotion got the better of me and I found myself shouting into the phone that warfarin would kill him quicker than any blood clot. It might surprise you to know that warfarin is the same product used in rat poison.

By the time I had booked my flight to come and see him, the emergency services had already been called. A team of paramedics were standing over his body trying to resuscitate him. Before I could even get on the plane, Dad's life had come to an abrupt end.

With no sign of life left in his body, the paramedics packed up their bulky equipment and left. Mom, of course, instinctively went back to holding his hand. Only after the warmth left his fingers did she think to call me long distance to deliver the bad news. With a great deal of dignity in her voice, she uttered these words, "I wanted to be the one to tell you that we lost Dad today."

Given his situation, I was expecting the call but it still hurt like a punch in the gut. A few days later I was back in the UK and saw my mom standing without her best friend for the first time. She did what all good moms do in the face of adversity of course and simply smiled through her pain.

For more than six decades, Mom cooked, cleaned and loved him. At the funeral, she looked like a butterfly trapped behind a pane of glass with no way out. And yet, she somehow found the strength to thank each and every person for coming. I now have a much deeper understanding of what the term "paying your last respects" really means.

Dad was ill and I accept that, and to be fair, everyone was doing the best they could in extremely difficult circumstances. But when six experts tell a human spirit that it's about to die, I believe that is what it does.

Like a small pilot light inside every one of us, the human spirit burns brightly wherever there is hope. It can accomplish things far beyond our understanding. But it can also be as delicate as a candle in the wind. Rest peacefully Dad, I'll miss your face and even your terrible jokes. I **hope** we'll meet again one day.

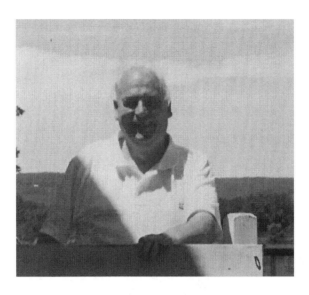

Hope is independent of the apparatus of logic. – Norman Cousins

Look, we all know this life isn't easy, even more so when we become ill. Trying to find answers when our world is falling apart can be a real challenge – believe me, I get it. But if you have made it this far in the book then you, like me, must have a knack for sticking with it. That takes guts, especially when you don't feel good, to begin with.

So here's my question to you: why are you still reading this book? What's driving you to keep going in the face of adversity?

I may not know you personally, but I suspect your inner spirit still burns brightly. This is actually a really good sign. Regardless of what's happening to your body today, you could be on the cusp of a unique turning point. At this point, I'd like to sincerely thank you for allowing me to be a small part of your journey. In case you didn't already know it, you are the reason I wrote this book. So keep coming, don't quit.

Okay, the second half of this book is about to kick off. Rest assured there are lots of fascinating new topics coming up. Rather than running out of steam, we are only just getting warmed up! As we move forward, I'll continue recommending good people to have on your team via the homework section.

What did we learn from this?
No matter what the world is throwing at you, your inner spirit appears to be intact. For anyone looking to overcome illness, this is an excellent sign.

Homework: If you want to go a little deeper with your learning then check out Mike Mutzel. Mike often chooses to interview those who are on the absolute cutting edge of natural medicine. Mike also has a degree in biology and has completed his M.S. in clinical nutrition from the University of Bridgeport. You can keep up to date by following him on Facebook. Here's the direct link for e-book users.

https://www.facebook.com/MikeMutzelMS/?hc_ref=ARQ1dAyhNhdQrz ldpZm66eiJtydtv5qjc1dLkRcW6S_i3p2J1q8C2hug1gvWhkMeDg8

Chapter 22

FIRST DO NO HARM

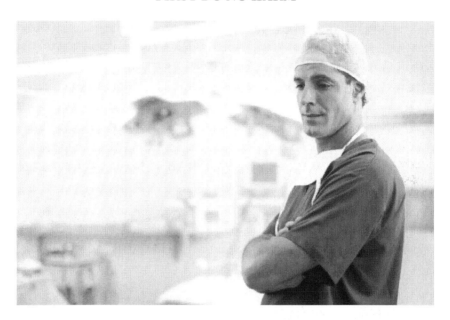

When it comes to broken bones, gaping wounds, heart attacks, or any type of sudden trauma the work a doctor does is nothing short of miraculous. These dedicated men and women deserve the highest credit and we should salute them for the brilliant work they do.

Good doctors listen to their patients and bring about good results — hoorah to all the good doctors! We should all be thankful to have them on hand when we need them. But that's not to say all doctors hit the same high standard.

The law of averages dictates that in any profession, from plumbers to brain surgeons, some folks will get the job done with speed and efficiency. Others? *Meh, perhaps not so much.*

Depending on your desire to get well, you may find stagnant results frustrating. If this is you, then rest assured, the gold standard for finding a good doctor is simple: if people are getting good results then they have a good doctor. If results are poor ...well, that's not hard to figure out.

That said, I don't believe any doctor goes to work with the intention of making mistakes. But when symptoms present themselves in a vague fashion, doctors may even fall short of our high expectations.

Let's remind ourselves that modern medicine still has a few things to figure out. Diseases such as chronic fatigue, crippling anxiety, and devastating depression continue to frustrate the medical profession. Cancer runs rampant and to date, we are still waiting for the elusive common cold cure. We could also add to the list more than a hundred debilitating autoimmune diseases. The root cause is often written off as either "unknown" or genetic.

There are times when medicine gets it right and, unfortunately, there are times when it gets it wrong. Doctors are not gods, with more than 400+ doctors committing suicide every year (in the US alone) I can assure you, they are just as human as you and I.

So the aim of this article is to guide you towards a good doctor. Although it's important to note that good doctors and nice doctors are not always the same thing. Here's a true story...

A friend of my family has been dealing with a health issue for the past year or so. She has worked in the medical industry most of her life and has a great relationship with the doctor treating her. It's obvious that she likes him (a lot) and she is now trusting him with her life. However, it's plain to see that twelve months into her illness, her progress has been stagnant. A more critical mind might suggest she has actually gotten worse.

We would do well to remind ourselves that any doctor we employ is there to fix a problem. As in this case, "nice" doctors have become better at public relations than they are at treating people.

If our goal is to get well, then look past the easy smile and cheery bedside manner and find someone with a proven track record. Even if that means you don't necessarily like the person or their methods.

LOOKING FOR A USED CAR?

So how do we set about finding a good doctor? That's easy, search for one with the same diligence we would when buying a used car. Before we step foot on a used car lot, most of us have done a little homework. We may have asked friends which cars they prefer and then cross-reference MPG ratings and prices etc. Some of us may even bring into question the car dealer's past integrity. And yet, when a car breaks down the only thing we stand to lose is a little money.

It displays an absence of sound reasoning to seek the services of a doctor without applying the same level of diligence. Using this simple technique, a motivated, informed patient should be able to spot an average doctor from a mile away.

Going into any new situation blind and expecting a positive outcome is at best hopeful. Prior to your appointment take notes and have a series of questions on hand. After a brief fifteen-minute appointment, don't be in a rush to hand over full responsibility for your health.

I'm rarely impressed with the bricks and mortar of a doctor's office or the fancy certificates on the wall. Rather, give me a doctor who can answer the "Why am I ill?" question. Pressing people for the cause of your illness allows you to evaluate that person's understanding of the problem. Without knowing the true cause, any treatment moving forward will be speculative.

It's important to be an active player in your own recovery. Let's stop blindly following the instructions of others in the hope that it's all going to work out for you. Come on now, deep down you know deep down I'm right. Some of us spend more time researching a vacation than we do a medical procedure.

So why is this so important?

The term medical malpractice is one we should ALL fear because it is now becoming a leading cause of death. If we break that down it simply means this: we go to the doctor, he or she gives us something for our illness, we take it, and we die.

No?

Okay, check this out.

In 1999 the pharmaceutical giant Merck released a drug by the name of Vioxx. With a TV budget running into the millions, Vioxx quickly became one of Merck's bestsellers. Americans were prescribed Vioxx as an aspirin substitute because it was believed to produce fewer complications. I know, right? What could possibly go wrong?

By 2007, people had begun to die and the class action suit that followed was eventually settled for $4.85 billion. But wait, there's more. By the time Merck paid its fine, it had technically made more profit from selling a deadly drug than it paid in fines! Conservative figures suggest that Vioxx killed hundreds, if not thousands of people, and yet nobody went to jail. What's up with that?

> Our prime purpose in this life is to help others.
> And if you can't help them, at least don't hurt them.
> – The Dalai Lama

The real concern is that Vioxx was first put on the market in 1999. Despite early alarm bells ringing Vioxx remained on the market right up until 2004! "First do no harm" is a noble oath that all good doctors aspire to; it's also the same one many of those doctors prescribing Vioxx took.

To expand on this point, we could easily use other examples of pharmaceutical drugs gone rogue, but I suspect you have already been conditioned to accept that side effects are a necessary evil. Just sayin, perhaps a doctors' iconic white coat should be required to carry the names of their sponsors the same way NASCAR drivers do.

Again, I'd like to be clear. Good doctors are out there, although it rarely bodes well to put our lives in their hands of someone we have only just met.

TRUE STORY

Clearly, things can and do go wrong with medical procedures, but for this next example imagine for a moment you woke one morning with serious pain in your left leg. Over time this pain worsened to the point where you began to use a wheelchair. As the pain intensified a friend quite rightly suggested that you see a doctor.

The news you received from the doctor is damning; tragically the doctor informs you that amputation is the only course of action. Despite reassurances that prosthetics have come a long way, you are deeply reluctant to cut off your left leg. On the way home your leg is hurting like hell and deep inside you accept that the doctor is right — obviously, that leg needs to come off.

A month or so later you find yourself back in the doctor's office flipping through a glossy prosthetic leg magazine. After filling out the paperwork you are relieved that a date has finally been set for the operation. Now imagine waking up from that same operation and seeing your idiot doctor holding up your right leg. Yes, he amputated the wrong leg. True story!

In 1995, Tempa surgeon Dr. Rolanda R. Sanchez of the University Community Hospital listed the wrong leg for amputation. He and his lawyer Michael Blazicek publicly presented their side of the story.

Personally, I would have thought it a difficult case to defend once exhibit "A" (the leg) was presented, technically leaving him without a leg to stand on, so to speak. Whoa! I'm just telling it like it is.

As for the patient, God only knows what he must have been thinking as he faced the unenviable decision of having to decide for a second time whether or not to have his left leg cut off.

But every cloud has a silver lining. The next time around we can safely assume that the chances our patient's correct leg will be cut off are as close to 100% as anyone could hope. Easy now … or would you rather I just deliver your medical news in a dull format?

You might think this is an isolated incident and you would be wrong. It is well documented that removing the wrong limb — and even the wrong organ — happens with disturbing regularity. During routine operations, there have even been reports of medical instruments gone missing and turning up stitched inside the patient!

My point is this: don't settle for average, do your research, be informed, fight your own corner or live with the consequences. Rushing into a relationship with a very nice but "average" doctor allows for ample opportunity to repent at leisure. If you are heading for a hospital, be sure to have good people around you and remain vigilant.

When faced with ANY invasive procedure first do your homework, speak to people who have been in your situation. Then compare their results with your expectations. People are always in a hurry to recommend nice people, but we should remember that we aren't looking for nice, we are looking for results.

Ultimately it's always going to be your health that's on the line. Hear me now, if something doesn't feel right with any procedure, speak up for yourself and politely but firmly say no. It's your body, which means you don't even have to explain yourself. You should never feel pressured to do something that makes you feel uncomfortable just to make someone else feel comfortable.

Good doctors aren't always the most expensive, nor do they need to have the best bedside manner. They do, however, have to have one dead giveaway. Good people are busy people, and that's okay if he or she brings results.

Try to keep this in mind. If you can pick up the phone and see the doctor (or dentist) the same afternoon, that should immediately be a red flag.

Most competent doctors will be booked solid as good news always travels fast.

If you can get in to see your doctor at the drop of a hat, then perhaps you should wait for that other guy. Obviously, this is subject to your appointment not being an emergency. In that case, you can rest assured that most ER doctors are nurses are some of the most efficient people on the planet.

Remember the golden rule. Whenever you meet a healthcare professional be polite and respectful but don't be afraid to ask probing questions. A good doctor/dentist will never feel threatened by an informed patient.

BLOOD WORK NUMBERS THAT DON'T ADD UP?

Finally, let's talk about blood work. In recent years' medicine has come to rely on a set of numbers as a way to diagnose illness. But there are lots of variables that aren't always taken into account.

The number a computer spits out for a 6' 5" man with green eyes shouldn't be in the same range as for a 5' 2" man with only one eye. *You catching ma drift?*

Sometimes the computer gets it right and sometimes it can give a false reading. But to a patient leaving a doctor's office with a set of blood-work numbers that don't stack up, it can become a source of great frustration. It's not uncommon for blood work numbers to say you are fine when you know deep down know you're not, and around and around in circles we go.

In days gone by, if a patient claimed to be unwell, then they were treated as being unwell. Today we appear to have this seemingly obvious truth a little twisted.

Old-school doctors would first ask a series of probing questions and then listened carefully to the answers. Today a computer is quick to churn out numbers based on averages. Essentially, a blood sample is attempting to make a match your blood with a patch of dry ink. This arrangement may work well for the computer, but let's not forget that we are humans, and our variables are often incalculable.

Am I saying blood tests have no place in medicine? Nope, never did say that. I'm saying it is imperative that you find a doctor who listens to you. The point I'm trying to drive home is this. To rely on a blood test while ignoring the patient has the potential to bend all the laws of common sense. And in doing so does a great disservice to the patient.

What did we learn from this?
The right doctor can be a godsend, but choose your new doctor/dentist with the same care you would choose a new (or used) car, and always do your homework. Ask questions and listen carefully to their answers.

Homework: find a good doctor to have on your team. If your circumstances allow it, you may find it helpful to search for someone who practices "Functional Medicine." As always, do your research to ensure you are in good hands.

Chapter 23

THE IMMUNE SYSTEM

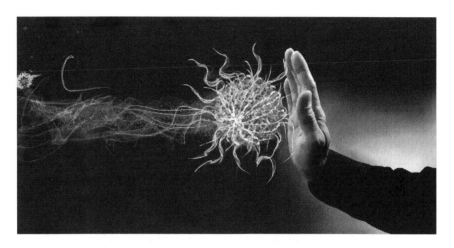

Ever see someone in the grocery store wiping "germs" off their shopping cart handle? I often wonder if those antibacterial wipes do little more than offer shoppers a false sense of security. *How so?*

Think about it, unless they are going to wipe the whole store down then where's the cutoff point? Does the farmer who picks the lettuce need to wipe down his hands? How about the guy loading the soda onto the truck? And the person cutting down bananas? How about the teen on summer break stocking shelves? If this is about "controlling" germs why don't the supermarkets offer wipes next to the credit card machine at the checkout?

Can you see where I'm going with this?

Unless we live inside a bubble it's impossible to control the environment around us. If the goal is not to get sick, then we have to control the environment within us.

For all my germaphobe homies out there, let's take this a step further. Many of those bacteria that freak you out so much are already living inside you. No really, it's true. Some estimates suggest they outnumber your cells by at least ten to one. Do the math, that makes us only ten percent human!

The trick to not getting sick is giving the immune system exactly what it needs. But there's more to boosting the immune system than meets the eye. If we look at the immune system under a microscope (these days that's pretty easy to do), we quickly realize that this system, above all others, is truly mind-blowing. Once fired up, the immune system is an equal match for a wide range of would-be enemies.

This formidable system can defend itself from multiple foreign invaders while at the same time, launching a counter-attack with deadly precision. To be clear—your immune system comes well-equipped to deal with high-level threats on a minute-to-minute basis.

But there is a problem, can you see it?

To keep your immune system running at optimal levels the body requires fuel in the form of key nutrients. Once found in abundance, many of these key nutrients are today missing from our food. In some cases, these nutrients have been replaced with toxic products in the form of processed foods sold to us by non-other than …. the same supermarket handing out those wipes! I know right, you couldn't make this stuff up.

For some of us, the immune system has now become a nutritionally downgraded version of its former self. Correcting the underlying nutritional deficiency would seem like a logical first step in the right direction. But that's not what many of us do.

> Thinking is difficult, that's why most people judge.
> – C.G. Jung

Rather than boosting the immune system with those missing key nutrients, we humans have taken this a step further by propping up a nutritionally downgraded immune system (AKA a weakened immune system) with pharmaceutical products.

For the past 100+ years, science has, with limited success, been locked in a bitter battle trying to rid the world of all infectious diseases. For the past fifteen years, that goal has somewhat intensified. And yet rates of serious illness continue to rise and nobody seems to know why. But there's another problem ..

Trying to control infectious diseases this way is like trying to squish a balloon. We eradicate one disease but then another pops up of greater magnitude. Autoimmune conditions can range from ALS to MS, from Type 1 diabetes to Rheumatoid arthritis, the list goes on and on and on. To date, a "confused" immune system can display itself in more than a hundred different ways! So with autoimmune conditions and counting, it begs the question … *Why?*

Why are rates of autoimmune conditions now skyrocketing? Could it be, in our relentless push to control "germs' we have reduced the risk of one illness but increased the risk of another? When the immune system is forced to deal with multiple weakened strains of diseases in one sitting are we running the risk of the immune system becoming hypersensitive or "confused"?

Perhaps this is the clearest signal yet that the man has underestimated the complexity of the immune system. I suspect there is more to this debate than meets the eye. But when the only tool being used is a hammer, everything begins to look like a nail.

This isn't a question of being for or against any particular ideology or practice. But when science tells us it doesn't know the reason behind autoimmune conditions then the door needs to open for debate.

Rather than becoming involved in a heated pro/anti debate, I'm simply suggesting we need to explore other pathways to fight disease. I believe one of those pathways is to remove anything of a toxic nature from the body (including excess sugar) and then flooding the cells with cutting-edge nutrition.

There's more than one way to skin a cat.
But from the cat's perspective, they all suck. – Ze-Frank

221

When the nutritional demands of the immune system are ignored, our quest to be disease-free has the potential to become a double-edged sword. As it stands, autoimmune conditions cost the economy billions of dollars each year, the cost in human suffering is incalculable.

The definition of an autoimmune condition is a system that has become confused to the point where it now fails to recognize the difference between itself and extensions of itself.

Once triggered, a confused immune system can launch an attack anywhere within. Having an autoimmune condition can be like having an octopus on your back. Its long tentacles reaching into every part of your body. Whatever it comes in contact with, it then attacks!

But the immune system is anything but dumb. When we treat it with respect it becomes a formidable ally. **Treat it wrong and you now have a highly complex problem that few understand.**

Make no mistake, autoimmune conditions are notoriously difficult to treat and just as tricky to diagnose. The moment your immune system turns rogue on you, doctors have little to offer in the way of permanent solutions. So how do you know if you have an autoimmune condition? That's easy, just answer yes to the six questions below.

1: Is your medical file as thick as the US tax code?

2: Have you seen three or more doctors in the last two years and yet you remain undiagnosed?

3: Do you have a cupboard full of medicine, but still feel ill?

4: Have you been told your bloodwork tests are "fine"?

5: Do you have a second cupboard full of natural supplements that appear to make things worse?

6: Adding insult to injury, somewhere along the way was it suggested that your suffering is all in your head?

If this is you, welcome to the perplexing world of autoimmunity!

It's widely believed that once you have one autoimmune condition the chances of getting a second begin to escalate. So, that's the good news out of the way. And now for the bad.

Once you have an autoimmune condition there is no cure for it; once the gene has been switched on it can't be switched off. However, before you throw yourself under a Number 52 bus, let me throw you a helpful lifeline. With the right tools, autoimmune conditions can be managed.

Food plays a huge role in this. No really, it's true. This would include restricting foods collectively known as lectins. A lectin free diet was recently brought into the mainstream by Dr. Gundy, a world-renowned heart surgeon. Dr. Gundy decided to switch gears and began using food as medicine. *Hmm, I see.*

Anyone with an autoimmune condition might find it helpful to excludes all grains, dairy (didn't we already cover these?), legumes, and foods belonging to the nightshade family. This would include foods like peppers, potatoes, and tomatoes. One way to reduce the lectin content of food is to cook those types of vegetables with a pressure cooker. The good news is, reducing lectins reduces symptoms.

Yup, it all takes effort, but once the immune system is brought back into balance symptoms can become minimal.

What did we learn from this?

Modern medicine is quick to point out that it doesn't have all the answers for this upsurge in autoimmune self-hacks, **which in turn should open the door for intelligent debate.** Alas, free thinkers are all too often demonized, categorized, and ultimately judged.

Chapter 23a

BONUS CHAPTER

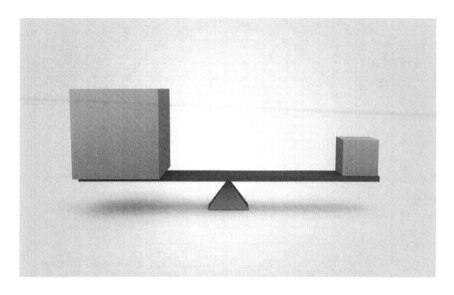

To help us understand what's happening on the outside, we first have to look on the inside. For this exercise lets split your immune system into two. We'll call the first half Th1 and the second half Th2. We'll then look deeper at the one that applies to YOU.

Ready?

Th, is an abbreviation for T-helper cells which form part of the immune system. Their job is to recognize and destroy any foreign microorganism that can cause disease. Th1 cells typically deal with infections by viruses and certain bacteria.

They are the body's first line of defense against any pathogen that gets inside our cells. Th1 cells tend to be pro-inflammatory. Th2 cells on the other hand typically deal with bacteria, toxins, and allergens. They are responsible for stimulating the production of antibodies. Th2 cells tend not to be inflammatory.

But what does that mean and why is this so important to know?

While it may sound complicated on the surface, it's really not. Both work sides of the immune system are working together, think of them as a kind of tag-team. Depending on the threat level, sometimes Th1 does more of the work and Th2 may play a lesser role. As the threat changes, roles are quickly switched. Once the threat has been neutralized the two stand down and return to equal balance. This is how a well-balanced immune system should work. **But there's a problem, can you see it?**

In an ideal situation, neither Th1 or Th2 is displaying a more dominant position. However, in some people, a prolonged pattern of either Th1 or Th2 dominance occurs and this is where health problems begin.

Knowing whether your immune system is Th1 or Th2 dominant plays an important part in the wellness puzzle. Not least because it allows you to figure out which is the best course of action to take (and which you should avoid!).

Perhaps now it makes sense why that cupboard full of natural supplements always makes you feel worse. Anything that boosts one side of the immune system tips the balance. Remember, balance is your body's preferred state.

SO HOW DO WE KNOW?

So how do we know if we are Th1 or Th2 dominant? That's a great question and the answer is relatively straightforward. For starters, there is a Th1, Th2 cytokine blood panel that your doctor can order.

Th1 cells are part of what's called cell-mediated immunity, which is an immune response that does not involve antibodies. It does, however, involve the release of various cytokines in response to foreign proteins. Let's simplify -if this problem was a basic image, this is how Th1 dominance might look.

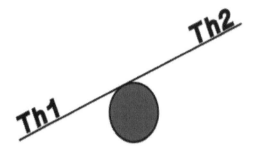

People who are typically Th1 dominant (but not all) may have delayed food sensitivities, increased brain fog, fatigue, increased likelihood of Type I diabetes, multiple sclerosis (although MS can be found in both Th1 and Th2 dominant types), Hashimoto's, Grave's disease, Crohn's Disease, psoriasis, Sjogren's syndrome, celiac disease, lichen planus, rheumatoid arthritis, and chronic viral infections. Again, these are generalizations and as with any autoimmune condition, it can easily manifest itself in multiple ways.

Being Th1 dominant means the immune system is constantly amped up. A telltale sign of the Th1 dominant person may be a tendency to catch fewer colds. Some reports even suggest lower cancer rates. But the devil is always in the details and as we mentioned earlier balance is super important. The downside of being Th1 dominant is a higher incidence of autoimmune conditions.

Th1 types should beware of any supplement that has the potential to boost the immune system. *Why?*

Supplements that increase Th1 also increase the problem. For example, natural supplements like Echinacea, astragalus, olive leaf, elderberry, and any medicinal mushrooms that are immune boosting. Be vigilant, because this is by no means a complete list!

NOW LET'S TAKE A CLOSER AT Th2 DOMINANCE

Having an immune system that is Th1 dominant is one thing but what happens when things swing the other way? Better hold onto your hat for a second, this is where it gets a little bumpy. *Ready?*

Functionally, Th2 cytokines have effects on many cell types in the body because the cytokine receptors are widely expressed in numerous cell types. Th2 cells stimulate and recruit specialized subsets of immune cells, such as eosinophils and basophils, to the site of infection or in response to allergens or toxins leading to tissue eosinophilia and mast cell hyperplasia. **I know, right? Who thinks this way?**

Let's look at an image of this instead. Ahhh, isn't that better?

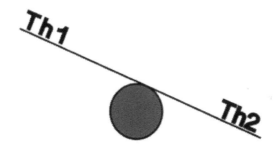

If we break this down into plain English, Th2 has some pretty beefy weapons called B cells and antibodies. These B cells are great to use in battle as they help produce more antibodies when needed. Essentially, this means they just keep on going and never run out of ammo—pretty cool, right?

This is done to ensure there is always enough ammo on hand should any foreign invader ever try to sneak into the body. Also, keep in mind that Th2 cells are anti-inflammatory.

227

Now, can you see the importance of a well-balanced immune system?

Once a foreign invader enters the body it becomes locked in battle with BOTH elements of Th1 and Th2. As the battle rages, the pro-inflammatory process needs to be "cooled down" using anti-inflammatory cytokines; hence it's a team effort. It's really not helpful having one side do all the work because left unchecked, systemic inflammation causes untold damage. When this form of inflammation is allowed to run rampant it can manifest itself in just ANY illness from headaches to cancer. It's the driving force behind every illness known to man.

When Th2 gets to be the dominant one, we may be more inclined to get seasonal allergies, asthma, food and drug allergies, and anaphylactic reactions rather than systemic inflammation. Th2 dominance can also be caused by a variety of issues such as heavy metals such as aluminum, mercury, and lead which are known to lower immune function. Heavy metals are such a fascinating topic that I'll cover it in more detail later. Okay, what else do we need to know?

When the immune system is shifted too much to the Th2 system, people generally have less inflammation but their potential to develop allergies to pretty much everything increases. It's the allergens that then begin causing problems.

Other possible diseases linked to Th2 dominant conditions may include Lupus, allergic dermatitis, atopic eczema, sinusitis, inflammatory bowel diseases, asthma, allergies, colitis, and multi-chemical sensitivities. Some reports even suggest an elevated Th2 may increase the risk of certain cancers. Either way, once the immune system gets stuck out of balance, we lose.

Interestingly, Lyme disease has the ability to throw Th1 out of balance because Lyme disease creates a state of perpetual Th1 dominance; this, unfortunately, results in constant inflammation, causing an ongoing downward spiral of damage in the body. *I know, right? Let's not go there, instead, let's focus on solutions.*

228

Because Th1 dominance is pro-inflammatory, we can now see the importance of eliminating all those foods that create inflammation. Foods loaded with preservatives, refined and fried foods, and fast foods all contribute to complicating the problem. But let's not forget our old friend sugar that can weaken the immune system and tip it out of balance.

Do you see how food keeps linking all this together? Spices like curcumin, turmeric, and ginger along with omega 3 oils are thought to be helpful because they may help counteract inflammation imbalance.

Th17

We seem to have covered a lot of ground here in one short read. In doing so I've attempted to keep the complex simple; (this is what I love to do most). However, the immune system is a vast subject and we didn't even get a chance to talk about Th17 cells. In case you are wondering why it's because they are a subset of activated CD4+ T cells that are responsive to IL-1R1 and IL-23R signaling. *I know, right? Just thinking about it gave me a headache too.*

However, if the whole Th1, Th2, Th17 concept has piqued your interest then continue reading. Autoimmune conditions are a tricky beast but I find them all rather interesting. If you would like to know more, please check out my book in today's homework section below.

LYMPH

Before we end I'd like to briefly mention the lymphatic system. As many may already know it's a network of tissues and organs that help rid the body of toxins, waste, and other unwanted materials.

The primary function of the lymphatic system is to transport lymph, a fluid containing infection-fighting white blood cells, throughout the body. Under each of your armpits (hello again) are more than twenty tiny lymph nodes. These small but highly sensitive lumps that act like tiny checkpoints. *But there's a problem, can you see it?*

The job of the lymphatic system's is an important one as it helps to fight infection. So you have to question the logic of squirting antiperspirant in such a delicate area. Especially when we stop and look at the loooong list of toxic ingredients (which usually includes aluminum). This can cause some people to sleepwalk into illness.

As the name suggests, antiperspirant stops your skin from perspiring by literally clogging it up. Seeing how the skin is the body's third kidney, it is alive and needs to breathe. With that in mind, perhaps applying an antiperspirant isn't a smart idea for anyone looking to overcome illness. The irony is the more we overload the lymphatic system the worse B.O becomes.

Unlike the heart, the lymphatic system has no pump and requires movement to push lymphatic fluid around the body. This fluid moves best when we move, which is more bad news if we happen to be sitting still most of the day squirting toxic chemicals under our armpits. The good news is, you don't need a gym membership to get the lymph moving. Hippocrates said it this way: "Walking is man's best medicine."

OO7

If walking isn't your thang, then my final tip for the day is to take a James Bond shower. This is effective at moving lymph and super easy to do. I just know you are going to love this one! First, hop into a hot shower and relax—feels good, right?

Now at some point simply turn the water all the way to cold and count to thirty, longer if you can stand it. Repeat this three times between hot and cold. This will help push the lymphatic fluid around the body. Doing it every day is no guarantee that you will live longer, but by the end of the week, it may seem like it, lol.

What did we learn from this?

The immune system works best when it is in balance. It's arguably the most complex, impressive, and effective system of all; it was put there to protect us. *Let's work with it, not against it.*

Homework: If this bonus chapter struck a chord with you, then a blood test may help uncover if you are Th1 or Th2 dominant.

You can also check out a website by the name of selfhacked.com. Here's the direct link: https://selfhacked.com As always *please feel free to mention where you found this information. Thanks.*

Chapter 24

A WALK ON THE DARK SIDE

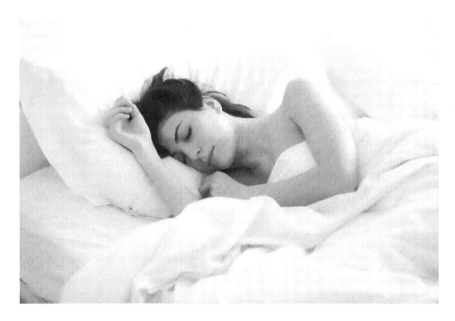

The better we sleep the better we feel. On the flip side, a lack of sleep can make us feel grouchy and run down. Our problem-solving skills decrease, reasoning becomes impaired, and attention to detail is lost. And yet, so many of us fight the idea of going to bed at a reasonable time. So the aim of this chapter is to first help you appreciate the value of your sleep and then show you ways to improve it.

Let's go take a look under the hood.

The brain gobbles up a whopping twenty percent of your daily energy! To be clear, your brain is an energy hog, even though it makes up only two percent of the body's weight. At night when you go to sleep, something remarkable happens. A cleanup crew gets to work and washes your brain to ensure that everything is ready for the next day.

It does this by using cerebrospinal fluid. This fluid is a clear liquid surrounding the brain and spinal cord. It moves through the brain along a series of channels that surround blood vessels.

This process is managed by the brain's glial cells. Science defines this as the "glymphatic system." It also helps to remove a toxic protein called beta-amyloid from brain tissue. Are you getting this? Sleep is kinda important. Beta-amyloid is known to accumulate in the brains of patients with Alzheimer's disease!

BRAIN DRAIN

From the moment your life began, the body has been using sleep to recharge and repair itself. We don't need to fully understand the mechanics; we just need to know that sleep can keep us healthy as well as assisting in any recovery.

In this digital age, we all grasp the importance of recharging our cell phones at night. And yet the brain uses more energy is infinitely more complex than any iPhone. So it shouldn't be surprising that our brain fails to work optimally when we fail to recharge ourselves with sleep.

TOCK-TICK

The sleep cycle begins as it starts to get dark outside, our brain then produces the hormone melatonin. This is how we evolved.
When morning breaks, light filters through the eye and melatonin production is switched off. But there's a problem, can you see it?

Today, our lives are impacted by the invention of the electric light. It's not a huge stretch of the imagination to think the electric light can have a similar effect as the daylight. More so if it has a blue hint to it which the brain may associate with the morning blue sky.

So this is actually quite simple. Our body is programmed to go to sleep when it gets dark outside and blue light can throw our sleep into total chaos. Altered melatonin levels have been linked to an increase in depression and irritability. Sabotaging your nighttime sleep with blue light is easy to do, it comes from our T.V screens, computers, LED lighting and video games. Hence, if we are looking for better sleep quality we need to begin shutting off these devices at least two hours before bedtime. If you want to become a champion sleeper, challenge yourself to become a total blue light Nazi.

Tip- You can limit the amount of blue light that's being emitted from your computer screen by installing a free app called F.lux. This tracks the time of day in your time zone. As evening comes around it gradually reduces the amount of blue light on your computer screen. It may seem a little odd at first, but it can serve as a helpful reminder that you should be winding down. If you decide you don't like it, simply uninstall it.

Light streaming in through a bedroom window is something else to think about. Street lights, car headlights, and even the moon can all affect your sleep. For better sleep, black-out curtains are an inexpensive fix. Obviously, if you find yourself waking in the middle of the night to use the bathroom be sure not to put those harsh bathroom lights on. Rather than disrupt melatonin, try using small plug-in night lights.

If you find yourself waking up in the middle of the night with a snack attack it could be a sign that your blood sugar isn't being regulated properly. If this is you, it may help to eat a bowl of rice an hour before bed. Although it's a carbohydrate, rice is pretty slow to digest.

If rice isn't your thang, try a teaspoon of raw local honey at bedtime instead, why? As you sleep, the brain still uses energy and does so by tapping into glycogen which is a form of sugar stored in the liver. If you try this route be sure to use locally sourced honey. Much of the honey found in the supermarket is imported; it's simply not the same standard as raw local honey and results will vastly differ.

It's also worth noting that caffeine is a stimulant that can stay in the system for six or more hours, even longer in sensitive people. Alcohol in the evening isn't going to help either. Initially, it may help you feel drowsy, but it will then prevent you from entering the deeper stages of sleep which is where the body does most of its healing.

If we are fortunate enough to live to the age of seventy-five, we will have spent, on average, twenty-five years of our lives asleep. Ever wonder what happens during that time?

When we lie down and close our eyes our brain rests and our heart rate slows. This restorative and relaxing part of sleep helps induce the NREM (Non-Rapid-Eye-Movement) sleep cycle. NREM sleep is then followed by the REM cycle (Rapid-Eye-Movement). Research has shown that REM is the part of the sleep that helps consolidate our emotions. This is also the cycle where muscles relax but the brain is in full activity.

As the name suggests, REM sleep is where our eyes begin rapidly darting back and forth. In this state, brain waves are most similar to our waking hours. This is deep sleep, but in order to get there, two things must happen. We need dark and we need quiet. Darkness helps with the production of melatonin and quiet just because I said so.

If you have been dealing with problems sleeping for any length of time, be sure not to take anything that might spook the system after 6 p.m. For sensitive people, certain medications and even supplements can throw sleep off.

I'm really not a fan of sleeping pills as they may leave a person feeling groggy throughout the following day. Even worse, drug dependence can become a problem down the road. If you need a little extra help to fall asleep try the following.

MAGNESIUM

Today it's not uncommon for people to have a magnesium deficiency. When this important mineral becomes depleted it can produce a wide range of serious ailments ranging from anxiety to cardiovascular disease.

Magnesium is used by the body as a currency for more than 300 enzymatic processes. Sustained levels of stress will often deplete magnesium levels. If our goal is to experience better sleep then magnesium is your friend.

However, before you head off to buy a bottle of magnesium pills please know that magnesium isn't absorbed very well through the digestive system. The better way to get magnesium into the system is by combining both oral and transdermal methods. Transdermal simply means that it is absorbed through the skin.

SALT AND SODA BATH

To increase your magnesium level (and help you sleep better), it may help to try a "salt and soda bath." To do this, simply pour a cup of quality Epsom salts into a hot bath one hour before bedtime and then soak in it. The heat will allow the Epsom salts to be absorbed through the skin and thus flood the system with magnesium sulfate.

Add the same amount of Arm & Hammer baking soda to the water and this may help drain the lymphatic system and balance your pH. Some reports suggest that a Salt and Soda bath may even be helpful to decrease radiation levels from x-rays—but that's a whole other story.

If salt and soda baths aren't your thing, you could try a transdermal magnesium. Simply apply to the skin throughout the day and then monitor how you feel. If the magnesium is of good quality, you can also expect to have more energy during the day and feel less stressed at night. Yup, magnesium really is that cool.

Without wanting to sound like a hippy, you could also add a few drops of lavender oil directly to your pillow. This will further aid relaxation and help reduce nighttime anxiety. This can be particularly helpful for young children. If you want to upgrade this technique try adding a few drops of lavender into an oil diffuser.

CBD

If you are still struggling to sleep, here's another tip you can try that's much safer than sleeping pills. CBD oil is taken directly on the tongue at bedtime and it gently eases us into sleep.

CBD oil has recently become more mainstream thanks to new numerous studies linking CBD oil to a wide range of health benefits. One exciting new study relates to children with uncontrollable epilepsy. In this area, CBD oil appears to be working where conventional medications have failed.

CBD oil is a legal derivative of cannabis; however, CBD oil can only be sold with the TCH component extracted. TCH is the part of cannabis that's sought after by people who are looking for a high. To be absolutely clear, CBD is a world apart from this. You cannot get high from CBD oil, sorry if that disappoints some readers.

BETA-1, 3D GLUCAN

If CBD oil still sounds a little too rock and roll for you then we could try something a little more traditional. With more than fifty years of research behind it, Beta-Glucans are arguably one of the most studied naturally derived supplements on the planet. Like so many other effective compounds, Beta-Glucans have a wide range of other benefits.

According to research carried out by Dr. Vaclav Vetvicka Ph.D., Beta-Glucan 1, 3D may even have some exciting cancer-fighting benefits. Today, we are looking only at its effectiveness as a sleep aid.

Beta-Glucans work as immunomodulators. This simply means it helps restore balance to the immune system. Think Th1 and Th2 imbalance from the previous chapter.

As with any product, you tend to get what you pay for. Beta-Glucans sold by Transfer-Point are a little more expensive than others but you may find them helpful. I have no affiliation with this company (or any other). If the price is an issue, don't be afraid to try some of the less expensive brands.

Sometimes it can be helpful to switch things around from week to week but it's important not to try too many things at the same time. A little tweaking on your part should put you on the right track. Just to be clear, I said tweaking not twerking.

There are lots of herbal teas to help you sleep and my personal favorite is chamomile tea. Allowing the tea to steep will increase its potency.

Another sleep hack to try is a grounding pillowcase. You can find these online. This pillow connects to the earth supply in your home and it may help to calm the mind. For it to work your home needs to properly earthed, you should obviously test this before buying the pillow. Testing can be done with an inexpensive tester from any DIY store; it's a light-up device and costs around five bucks.

There are plenty more sleep hacks to try, but rather than overwhelm you, remember that we don't want to try them all at the same time. Better to start small and see how you feel, using too many things at once is always counterproductive.

Many of us have heard that we need a standard eight hours of sleep, but the quality of sleep is important. I'd like to suggest that we all have different needs, some of us may do better on six hours of sleep and others may need more.

Ever wonder why teenagers always seem to need more sleep? The teenage years are a critical time for brain development. It's unfortunate that teenagers, who have the most need for sleep, are often the ones who don't get enough.

Perhaps we should be encouraging them to sleep in more, not less. If you are a teenager, show this book to Mom; if you are a mom, let your teenager know playing grand theft auto at midnight isn't helping the cause. Perhaps a trade could be an early night off the computer for a few hours of extra sleep in the morning.

What did we learn from this?
Without sleep life quickly becomes dull and stressful. Sleep is an essential part of living which is why we typically spend a third of our lives doing it. Blue light at night is a huge problem as it throws our whole system out of whack.

Homework: here's a real moving TED Talk by a dad with a pot-taking eleven-year-old daughter. I know right, but this talk will totally challenge your perspective on CBD oil.

It's called "Why I changed my mind about medicinal cannabis" by Hugh Hempel. E-book readers can simply click on the link below.

https://www.youtube.com/watch?v=3N8QMeIsX2c

Chapter 25

WHERE TO FIND THE CLEANEST FOOD

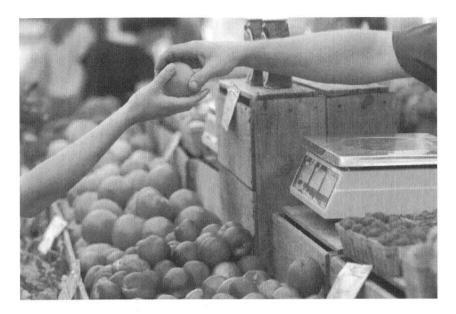

During the 1950's my grandparents owned a thriving fruit and vegetable shop in the North of England. With the exception of a few non-GMO bananas, everything they sold had been grown within a ten-mile radius. Out of pure economic necessity, what came and went through their front door was local, sustainable and in season.

Back in the day, this was just how food was traded. Fast forward to today and the words "local and organic" have suddenly become lucrative buzzwords. I'm pretty sure if my grandad were still alive he'd be left scratching his head knowing that the business model he once used out of pure necessity, would today be seen as trendy or even upmarket. Here's where the story gets interesting.

Bugs eat profits. I know this and so do large-scale organic farmers. Make no mistake, farming is hard work and you can bet anyone getting up at 5 a.m. is in it to make money like everyone else. And to be clear, there is nothing wrong with making money at 5 a.m. or any other time of day. However, if you think all your organic produce arrives at your table pesticide free you are wrong. Large-scale organic farmers aren't about to risk crop failure and certain financial ruin just to bring you a fresh head of kale.

Ever wondered why your organic kale comes to the table without hundreds of tiny bug holes in it? It's been sprayed with an "organic" pesticide. What you need to quickly wrap your head around is that ALL pesticides, organic or not, share a common goal: to repel living things.

According to the USDA, the organic label only restricts the use of synthetic pesticides. Pesticides like copper sulfate and rotenone are permitted to be sprayed directly onto your organic produce. Am I saying don't buy organic? Nope, that's not what I am saying at all, but some of us have become so desperate to believe in the benefits of organic food that we only see what we want to see. The aim of this chapter isn't to tickle your ears with sweet words, it's to help you understand the value of clean, local food and show you where to find it.

Not all organic food is as squeaky clean as we would like it to be. With that in mind, perhaps some of the smaller local farmers without an organic seal are being harshly overlooked.

BIG PHARMA — LITTLE FARMER

Let's take this a step further by looking at that pristine organic USDA seal of approval. Would it surprise you to know that it can be handed out to products that use only 95% organic ingredients during processing? For this reason, anything carrying the organic label may not be strictly 100% organic.

Look, I'm not shooting organic food down — I'm simply saying that in today's busy world of commerce it pays to be aware that the only truly organic food is homegrown. Your next best option is to know the name of the farmer who grows it.

The controversy over organic food can begin even before the first seed is planted. Whether or not the seeds are organic means only one thing: that the original seed-producing plant was grown according to organic standards. If a hybrid seed is planted, the resulting plant will still be organic so long as synthetic pesticides and fertilizers aren't used.

To be clear, organic food that's been grown specifically for supermarkets has its place in your recovery. It's a huge step in the right direction and an absolute upgrade of what they usually try to sell us. The point I am trying to make is this: don't be too quick to discount your small local farmer just because he/she doesn't carry that holy grail of organic seals.

Try looking at it this way: there was a time when our ancestors' food was truly organic. Today farmers who choose to grow "organic" food are often shackled in regulation. The irony is those nonorganic farmers who drown our foods with synthetic pesticides are less regulated.

Surely we have this all twisted. Shouldn't the regular farmers who are spraying copious amounts of carcinogenic pesticides on our food be the ones held accountable and buried in paperwork?

Either way, there are times when small independent farmers can't get the organic certification simply because of the added paperwork and costs involved. Fees typically include paying the government for site inspections, application fees, and annual certification fees.

If an organic farmer wishes to conform to all the regulations he/she must find the time to stop work whenever a government bureaucrat visits the farm. If the small local farmer wants the organic seal, he/she is inevitably forced to jump through hoops to get it and in the process loses valuable time and resources. With the small local farmer now squeezed out, I sometimes feel we are quick to trust the large-scale organic label and slow to ask questions.

As evolutionary biologist Christie Wilcox explained in a 2012 Scientific American article, even "organic" pesticides can be toxic. Copper sulfate, when digested in large amounts, can lead to damage in the tissues, blood cells, liver, and kidneys. While I'm not suggesting toxic levels are being applied, we should be aware of any pesticide that has the potential to cause us harm.

Rotenone is another pesticide sprayed onto organic crops and is notorious for its lack of degradation. Studies show that copper sulfate, pyrethrins, and rotenone can all be detected on plants after harvest. Hmm, I see, perhaps we need ask more questions of large-scale farmers, not fewer.

With (or without) the government organic seal of approval, enthusiastic young farmers are the lifeblood of the local food movement. They often bring clean food to farmers' markets and shouldn't be discredited for lack of paperwork.

Diversity in farming is a good thing and relying too heavily on a small number of people for our food should be an obvious cause for concern. Many small farmers are the backbone of independent farming and they deserve your support just as much as any large-scale organic farmer does.

The goal of this chapter isn't just to get you to buy clean food, I'm asking you to go a step further and know the name of the farmer who grew it! Make a connection with the person growing your food. Small farmers need you to survive and you need them to thrive. Ask yourself, how many of your friends on Facebook are farmers?

Still not convinced, huh?

Imagine we find ourselves stranded on a desert island with 150 other people and one bag of seeds. Everyone agrees that three things are needed for our survival: food, water, and shelter. Fortunately, this island currently has enough coconuts to get us through the first few weeks while the (non-GMO) seeds grow. Unfortunately, nobody seems to have a plan beyond this so the group decides to put YOU in charge of its survival. I know, right? Now we are all up the creek without a paddle.

You quickly realize that you need to make some pretty big decisions. What percentage of this group will you send out to find water? How many do you put in charge of growing those seeds? How many do you put to work building a shelter? If you split the group evenly into 50–50–50, I think you'll eventually be okay.

Even if you split the group 20–70–60 I still think you will make it. However, if you choose to have 149 people sitting around looking at computer screens all day while just one person grows the food, I'll think you are certifiably insane.

How is this relevant?

It should make you feel a little uneasy to know that, statistically speaking, the U.S. has just one farmer responsible for feeding 155 people seven days a week. This situation becomes a little more unnerving when you understand that most supermarkets have an inventory strategy called JIT (Just-in-Time).

Supermarkets employ JIT to increase efficiency and decrease waste by receiving goods only as they are needed. Even a small disruption in the JIT supply would see our supermarket shelves quickly stripped bare.

Are we there yet?

No?

Okay, try this. With or without an organic seal, small local farmers have a passionate connection to their land — it's in their blood. Local produce is always fresher from the local farmer and often less expensive. Superstores are now growing at an expediential rate with some of them now opening around the clock seven days a week, taking with them a huge slice of independent pie.

When the purchasing power of superstores is allowed to become disproportionately influential, income is taken away from the surrounding local businesses. When all the small businesses are gone, giant superstores will be free to dictate what you eat so long as it remains profitable for them to do so.

245

Fortunately, superstores are not the only game in town and you can still find clean food locally in small mom and pop shops or at your local farmers' market so long as we get out there and support them. Buying food locally also gives you the added benefit of buying what's in season and fresh.

Compared to the huge superstores (which never seem to close) small farmers' markets are usually held just once a week, obviously reducing their competitiveness with the bigger players. Unless we get out and support them more, this way of trading food will soon vanish.

What's in it for you?

I know you've been paying attention, so you already know the key to your recovery is your gut. It takes whatever nutrients you give it and then loops it back into the cells. Rather than buying your "organic" broccoli from a superstore, when you buy local you actually get to meet the person growing it. Where there is a connection there is also accountability.

Am I saying you have to cut the giant superstores completely out of your food loop? Nope, but it's important we try to adjust the balance by sourcing as much locally grown produce as possible. I get it, waiting once a week for a farmers' market can increase your chances of going without, so rather than complaining about it don't be afraid to take a shopping list with you on farmers' market days. But why stop there?

Once you have made a connection with your local growers it's totally okay to ask them if you can buy from them directly on non-market days. Often small local farmers will have additional eggs, vegetables, and meat for sale and they may even be pleased that you asked.

This is how food used to be bought and sold. Sometimes you just have to open your mind and be on the lookout for nutritional opportunities rather than following what everyone else does.

Having a thriving farmers' market in every town used to be the norm, but what can you do if your town or city doesn't have one? The most obvious choice is to move. Yup, finding clean food obviously needs to become a bigger priority in your life. Failing that, I encourage you to travel to the next town or to the one after that. You could also think outside the box and approach your local supermarket produce manager and ask if he or she would consider carrying more local produce. This idea supports your local farmer and it may be a good fit for all concerned.

If you still can't find a local farmer, then you could try hooking up with a local gardener. Anyone who grows food for a hobby usually grows more than they need. Generally speaking, gardeners are a pretty friendly bunch and they enjoy doing what they do — it's why they do it. Who doesn't like to have their hobby appreciated?

If your budget is ultra-tight, keep a lookout for garden allotments. This untapped idea can be a nutritional goldmine. This leads me nicely into the suggestion that even if you only have a small window box, you can begin to grow something yourself. This won't sustain you, but it does serve as an important psychological step to get you thinking differently about local food.

> Growing your own food is like printing your own money.
> – Rod Finley

People often complain about the price of clean produce, which is why our ancestors played a much bigger role in growing their own. Today you can still buy a pack of 250 organic lettuce seeds for a few bucks. A single fully-grown store-bought lettuce will cost you more. Lettuce seeds are super easy to grow and even when left unattended they grow like weeds.

The same applies to tomatoes. You really don't need much skill or more than a couple of feet of soil to grow them in. I agree it all takes time, but so does checking your email.

Once you see how easy it is to grow a few lettuces and tomatoes you may even become bold enough to grow even more things for yourself.

We spend millions of dollars keeping our lawns green, yet you can't eat the stuff and you certainly can't smoke it. Growing something, anything, that gets you thinking beyond the scope of the supermarket.

These superstores have become masters of distraction and even with the best intentions, we keep finding ourselves going back into them for organic food and leaving with a pair of socks. Think about it, these distractions put your food bill up every time you go to the store.

Perhaps we need to look at this problem from a different perspective. In Sweden, a small group of city folks took it upon themselves to grow just a few basic vegetables. At the end of the growing season, they traded with each other for more variety. It worked out well for everyone involved. So why does this feel so unnatural to us?

A little more food for thought (author knuckle bumps reader for unintended pun): imagine if one day visitors from another galaxy dropped in to visit and began observing those crazy Swedes growing their own food.

They then observed that other group, yup, you know who I mean, the ones being slowly poisoned to death by pesticides. Which group would the aliens regard as crazy? The group of humans working together to grow what keeps them alive, or the group of humans eating out of cardboard boxes while sitting on their excessively manicured lawns?

So, while we are waiting for our home-grown lettuce to come to fruition let's ponder our options. They say the road to hell is paved with good intentions. Promises and plans must be put into action, otherwise, they are useless. The way to make this work is to make the small local stores your first port of call and then fill in any gaps at the supermarket. Doing it the other way around rarely happens.

In all sectors, diversity is the lifeblood of healthy commerce; whether you are buying a cabbage or a carpet, small family business owners need our support.

After both of my grandparents passed away, the fruit and veg shop quickly changed hands. Today it sells bargain-priced booze and the only place to buy fresh produce is at the giant supermarket down the road. Perhaps as a reflection of our changing times, all the supermarket vegetables come tightly wrapped in plastic. Quite remarkably, it is estimated that those same vegetables will have traveled an average of 1500 miles to get to the supermarket. I know, right? It kinda makes a mockery of the whole cutting carbon emissions thing.

Without economic diversity, the world would become a very scary place. I'm reminded of how the Cadbury company once managed to successfully run their chocolate empire with exemplary values. Today? Meh, not so much.

From humble beginnings, Cadbury's chocolate began in 1824 by a family of practicing Quakers. As they grew so did their workforce. As a way of giving back to the local community, workers were taken out of dirty slums and moved into houses built expressly for Cadbury employees in a beautiful village environment.

At a time when many workers were uneducated, Cadbury also built a school for its employee's children and a doctor's office where Cadbury workers could receive free medical care. Mr. Cadbury regularly walked the factory floor and not only knew the names of his workers, he knew the names of their family members. The Cadbury workforce had value and working conditions steadily improved year after year.

Throughout Victorian times, the Cadbury name continued to grow, in part thanks to a loyal workforce. The Cadbury brand prided itself on selling only quality products. As the business expanded, it was suggested that growth could only be sustained if the Cadbury family began to advertise. A meeting was set up and several ideas were pitched to the Cadbury owners.

After several hours, all the ideas were rejected on the grounds that it was dishonest to suggest their chocolate product was better than it was.

Fast forward and today the Cadbury chocolate company is no longer in the hands of the Cadbury family. Instead, it was broken up and sold. I suspect some of the new owners never set foot on the factory floor.

While the price of the company may have increased in value, the value of a Cadbury worker has never been more undermined. When American food giant Kraft moved in to buy up the Cadbury brand, workers were seen protesting with banners that read, "Please don't sell us out." Today it seems the value of those workers is secondary to the profit line.

> Try not to become a man of success,
> but rather try to become a man of value.
> – Albert Einstein

What did we learn from this?
On average, just one farmer is responsible for growing the food of approximately 155 people. Buying local produce in season will enhance your nutritional intake as well as help the local community grow. Small independent shops often have greater ties with local growers which helps keep the local cycle going.

Homework: Challenge yourself to know the name of your local farmer. Find a farmers' market in your area and support it. Next, grow one thing from seed and see where it leads.

Check out this video from Dr. Axe
 https://www.youtube.com/watch?v=TUMNYkdxc9s

Paperback homies can Google "11 steps to losing belly fat by Dr. Axe."

It's worth noting that although Dr. Axe offers nicely packaged information that is easy to follow, you can also expect to find a few of his products being sold.

Chapter 26

TRICKY FOOD TRIGGERS

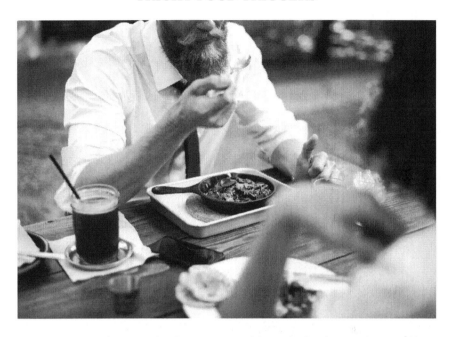

Straight out of the gate the four most problematic foods are gluten, dairy, eggs, and nuts, closely followed by corn. Having this vital piece of information early will serve us well as we move through the rest of this article. That said, the list of foods known to trigger a reaction is long and varied. As surprising as this may sound, many trigger foods are perceived to be healthy. To be clear, organic food has the potential to act as a trigger with the same intensity as its nonorganic counterpart. *No really, it's true.*

I know what you are thinking because I've had the same thought—why would the immune system react like this to healthy organic food? First, let's first back up and get a better understanding of what a reaction is and *isn't.*

To describe any reaction to food, you may hear terms such as a food intolerance, food allergy, and food hypersensitivity. Often times they are used interchangeably. This is not only confusing, it's also incorrect. *Here's why.*

Food intolerances are relatively common and are said to affect one in five of us. Reactions can vary, but the immune system is not involved in a food intolerance. Trying to replicate a reaction to a known food intolerance is difficult. Not least because there can be any number of factors that contribute to the intolerance. Food intolerances are known as non-immunological reactions.

By comparison, food allergies or hypersensitivity are a reaction to a protein found in certain foods. This does involve the immune system. This type of reaction is less common and is believed to affect one in fifty of us.

The good news is, once we learn to recognize the connection between food and the way it makes us feel, it becomes an empowering tool. And here's the not so good news.

Once the offending protein has been identified, a predictable reaction can then be replicated. With some degree of certainty, even a small amount of problem food will cause a reaction by the immune system. These types of reactions are known as immunological reactions.

As soon as your body has labeled a particular food as problematic, antigens are then made that ignite the immune response. Antibodies that bind to those antigens are then formed. To simplify, we could think of this process as the body highlighting any foreign invader it deems suspect. The body does this as a way to guide an attack by the immune system. So that the science bit out of the way but we still need to know why the immune system is doing this in relation to food.

To better understand, know that you aren't the only one who likes to eat — so do bugs. Certain plants already know this, but they can't exactly pick themselves up and run away. To keep themselves from being eaten alive, they have learned to adapt. Some plants now have the ability to produce small amounts of reactive chemicals. Depending on how sensitive your digestive system is, some people will react more violently to these chemicals than others.

NIGHTSHADES

Food in the nightshade family can cause a wide range of problems. It's worth noting that there are more than 2000 plants in the nightshade family. Thankfully, the list of the ones you might want to eat is relatively short, here it is.

• Tomatoes

• Tomatillos

• Eggplant

• White Potatoes (but not sweet)

• Goji Berries

• Peppers (bell peppers, chili peppers, paprika, tamales, tomatillos, pimentos, cayenne etc.)

• Tobacco (some people chew it)

Foods in the nightshade family are thought to weaken the tight joints in the small intestine. (Hello again cheeky-leaky gut). This allows tiny food particles (and excrement) to spill into the bloodstream. Now we have our trigger, we also get an increased hit of inflammation, I'll go over inflammation in more detail later. For now, I want to keep our wellness puzzle neat and tidy and running in logical order. Hence the topics we have already covered are now beginning to make sense.

The good news is if you commit to cutting out foods in the nightshade family you can expect to see an improvement in symptoms. Those symptoms may include (but are not limited to) joint pain such as arthritis, fatigue, and muscle pain and tightness. Are you catching this joint pain sufferer?

If this is you, try eliminating foods in the nightshade family for 30 days and watch what happens. A quick word of warning, this isn't something you can do halfheartedly. *Why?*

Once the immune system has been spooked, it's always on red alert. This means you can't cheat even a teeny weeny little bit. Everywhere you go, so does your immune system. This is something to be mindful of particularly if you don't feel well after eating. Geesh, do you see how this is all beginning to link together?

Unfortunately, foods that are capable of triggering an adverse reaction aren't confined to the nightshade family. As we have some ground to cover let's leave nightshades for the moment and take a closer look at types of food mold.

MOLD

In one form or another, we are all exposed to low levels of food mold. This isn't just the mold we see growing on stale bread. It's often too small to see with the naked eye and just about any food is susceptible. There is a school of thought that suggests that a peanut allergy may in part be due to the mold found on peanuts. While the nut debate remains speculative, I thought it an interesting addition to the subject.

In sensitive individuals, repeated exposure to any kind of food mold will make the diagnostic process quite challenging. Hence once again, awareness becomes key. Low-level exposure to food mold can present itself as headaches or brain fog. Higher levels can result in more serious problems.

With so many everyday foods prone to mold, even coffee can become a culprit. EU countries, South Korea, and Japan have strict regulations regarding levels of mold found in coffee. Ironically, in the U.S. and Canada, there are no such limits. *What's up with that?*

If you are a coffee drinker, be sure to get your coffee as a whole bean and grind it up yourself. Beans with the least amount of mold often come from the higher elevations. I'll take more about this later and I think you are going to be pleasantly surprised.

LECTINS

Lectins are extremely problematic for anyone with a suspected autoimmune condition. Although you may not have heard of lectins, scientists have known about them since 1884. Lectins are found in abundance in certain fruits, vegetables, beans, nuts, legumes, milk, and members of the yup, they are also in the nightshade family (and hello again to you Mr. potato).

Lectins (not leptins) are a type of protein that can bind to cell membranes. They are sugar-binding and become the "glyco" portion of glycol-conjugates on the membranes. Some research suggests that cutting out lectins can reduce autoimmune symptoms to the point where they become manageable.

There are literally thousands of versions of lectins but not all of them are truly problematic. The ones that are capable of causing any irritation to the gut lining are the ones to watch out for. The worst offenders, deemed to have vastly higher lectin contents are listed below.

FOODS HIGH IN LECTINS

• All grains and cereals

• Nightshades, including tomatoes, peppers, potatoes, and eggplant

• Gluten from wheat, rye, barley, malt. (Maybe even oat on occasion because of cross-contaminated during processing)

• Beans and legumes, including soy and peanut. Cashews are considered part of the bean family

• All dairy, including milk, cheese, cottage cheese, yogurt, and kefir

• Yeast (except brewer's yeast and nutritional)

• To be on the safe side, fruits should be restricted during the first 30-day trial period and then gradually reintroduced.

For whatever reason, some people are more likely to have sensitive reactions to lectins than others. In most cases, seeds can be notoriously hard to digest. Perhaps mother nature constructed them that way to ensure that any animal eating the seed will later poop it out intact. For we humans, soaking seeds until they sprout a tail can help with digestion.

Foods with lower levels of lectins include mushrooms, broccoli, onions, bok choy, cauliflower, leafy greens, pumpkin, squash, sweet potato, carrots, and asparagus, as well as berries, citrus fruits, pineapple, cherries, and apples.

You can also add to this list animal protein from fish, seafood, eggs, meat, and poultry, as well as fats from olive oil, avocado, and butter — all of which have low levels of lectins. Before you throw yourself under a number 53 bus, know that you can reduce your overall lectin intake by cooking with a pressure cooker, I'll touch on this again later. Moving along nicely, let's take a closer look at grains capable of triggering the immune system.

GRAINS

Today, grains are found in everything from pasta to spice mixes, cakes to processed meats, and even salad dressing. The list is impossibly long so it's important to note that they can be found in just about any subset of food. Because of the way grains are stored when harvested, they can also be susceptible to hidden molds. For some, any grain can become a problem but the one I'm sure you have already heard of is gluten.

While some people may believe that going gluten-free is some kind of new fad, the discovery of this problem grain was actually first made in Holland by professor Willem-Karel Dicke back in the early 1950s.

Gluten is the seed of wheat and an insoluble protein composite. In plain English, this simply means it's difficult for the digestive system to break down. If I were a betting man (which I'm not), I'd bet that grains are, at least in part, contributing to most of the symptoms in the gut. "All Disease Begins in The Gut." — Hippocrates.

As mentioned earlier, an intolerance to gluten isn't the same thing as an allergy. An intolerance is the lesser of the two evils and it can certainly rear its head in any number of ways. But comparing a gluten intolerance to an allergy is the equivalent of comparing a very bad sunburn to a third-degree burn.

A true allergy to gluten becomes a more serious autoimmune condition known as celiac disease. This results in damage to the small intestine whenever gluten is ingested.

A common mistake people often make when they are told they have an issue with gluten is they then load up on gluten-free bread or gluten-free cookies. But, wait, that's good, right? Meh, not so fast.

Once you have a problem with gluten you have a spectacularly higher probability of reacting negatively to other grains. Simply switching to a different grain that doesn't contain gluten is like switching to a different pack of cigarettes.

Some people have an immediate and noticeable reaction to gluten; others have a delayed reaction that can occur gradually over several days. This type of disconnect becomes more challenging to deal with.

If you suspect you have a problem with gluten, the easiest way to test it is to go totally grain free for thirty days. After thirty days, watch what happens as you reintroduce grains into your diet. Yup, you could also get tested by your doctor, but any treatment is going to involve a strategy of total avoidance.

You might wonder why gluten is suddenly getting so much heat when bread dates back to biblical times. That's a nice thought and I'm going to award you five points for effort. But you are perhaps thinking of wheat as being three feet tall and blowing gently in the wind. *Am I right?*

Sadly, those types of romantic golden wheat fields are long gone. They have been replaced by a much smaller, genetically modified version. To add to the problem, this type of wheat is often soaked with a broad-spectrum systemic herbicide known as glyphosate (Roundup). Is it me, or is Roundup beginning to cause more problems than it was intended to solve?

We could easily fill up the rest of our time together talking about problems relating to glyphosate and gluten. But for simplicity's sake, let's agree that for many, gluten avoidance has the potential to bring huge health benefits.

However, to do this right, we need to stop looking at this as being gluten-free and go completely grain free. This is the single biggest reason people with gluten problems fail to see progress.

Tip — To help you on your way, check out a book called Against All Grain by Danielle Walker. It's packed with good ideas and healthy recipes.

CHECK IT

Below is a list of foods believed to cause approximately 90% of all food allergies. Take a look and ask yourself which of these foods you consume on a regular basis?

Wheat and other grains with gluten, including barley, rye, and oats

- Milk and milk related products, yogurt, and cheese

- Eggs

- Peanuts (prone to molds)

- Tree nuts, like walnuts, almonds, pine nuts, brazil nuts, and pecans

- Soy

- Fish (mostly in adults)

- Shellfish (mostly in adults)

- Food additives

Finally, I'd like you to hear the remarkable story of Dr. Terry Wahl's.

Dr. Wahl's was once a patient with a chronic, progressive disease and found herself confined to a wheelchair. As a qualified doctor, she used all her medical connections to the fullest. Even so, her condition got steadily worse.

In desperation, she tried a new path that included avoiding certain trigger foods. Today she walks free. Coming from a doctor I found her TED Talk fascinating and it's in today's homework.

What did we learn from this?
Once you have a spooked immune system, food can become an exploding minefield. To complicate matters, some of these trigger foods are often perceived as being healthy organic foods.

Homework: listen to Dr. Terry Wahl's TED Talk. If you are reading the paperback version of this book, a simple Google search will take you there. It's called "Minding your mitochondria" Enjoy.

https://www.youtube.com/watch?v=KLjgBLwH3Wc

Chapter 27

THE WORLD WE LIVE IN

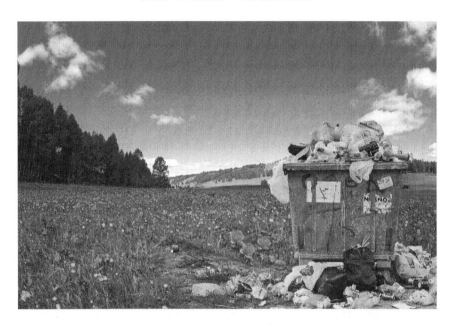

Over the course of a lifetime, it's estimated that the average American will purchase his or her way through a cool 2.7 million dollars' worth of stuff. If owning more stuff enhances your life, then more power to you.

But at some point, all that "stuff" will need to find a way back to the same earth it came from. So take a look around, is stuff really making you happy or has it become a ball and chain around your neck?

As you read this article, try to keep in mind that many of us drive around with more spare change in our cars than many people live on per day. And yet, some of the brightest smiles come from people with the least possessions? What's really going on here? Why are they so happy and how does any of this affect you? Let's take a closer look.

According to American credit card statistics, in 2015 the average US household carried $15,675 in credit card debt and $132,158 in total debt.

That's a lot of stuff, and potentially a whole lot of stress. Did I mention that stress is a killer yet?

People now own so much stuff they can no longer fit it all inside their houses. It has to be stored out in a shed, over in the barn, crammed into the attic or stuffed in the basement. And when all those places are full, the trend now is to rent a storage unit! FFS how much stuff do we really need?

Wait a second, didn't Gordon Gekko, the lead character in the classic movie Wall Street, once tell us that greed is good? Huh … really? With rising sea levels and darker environmental skies, maybe that classic line from Wall Street should have been "The highest wealth is the absence of greed." — Seneca:

This planet that feeds you, your children, and your grandchildren can sustain us all. It just cannot sustain the current rate of consumerism. The key to solving this problem is never going to be more recycling. Lord knows we've tried that and recycling more plastic really is one of man's dumbest inventions, here's why.

The average chunk of plastic can take up to 450 years to decompose. And yet we continue to produce single-use plastic bags, straws, coffee cup lids and water bottles in mind-boggling quantities.

Last year Americans drank their way through 50 billion water bottles (that's billion with a B). But here's the kicker, the US recycling rate is a mere 24%, which means 38 billion water bottles suddenly became someone else's problem.

Are you catching this? - It's kinda important.

Each time you place that discarded plastic item into your wheelie-bin, so do your friends, your family and all of your neighbors. This continues to play out until the system becomes totally flooded with plastic.

Wealthy nations then resort to paying poorer nations to take their unwanted plastic. No really, India has a growing mountain of the stuff.

So on the surface recycling may seem like the honorable thing to do, but at best, it's indirectly, feeding an insatiable commercial beast. At worst it's exploiting others into dealing with our waste.

> Treat the earth well: it was not given to you by your parents, it was loaned to you by your children- ancient American proverb

This really isn't rocket science, it takes energy to manufacture plastic just as it takes energy to recycle it again, thus ensuring the planet is having to work twice as hard. But if you stop and think about it, the plastic industry only exists because there is a demand. Take away the demand and you take away the need to recycle. It's a revolutionary idea I know, but the greenest of all plastic is the plastic we don't use. But there's more to this story than meets the eye.

There's always been an emotional "feel good' factor to placing our unwanted packaging into the recycling wheelie bin (phew, the planet gets to live another day), but in the real world, plastic is still getting dumped into the sea every minute of every day. Some estimates suggest that by 2050 there will be more plastic in the sea than there are fish!

But why should you care?

Well, packaging is just packaging until money changes hands and then it turns into pollution. We all like to drink clean water, breathe fresh air, and look at the big blue sky, *am I right?*

I know what you are thinking because I had the same thought. Pollution is China's problem, right? Sadly, pollution has an uncanny knack for being whipped up into the jet stream. What goes up must come down which is usually thousands of miles away from where these toxic goods were made. But there's a bigger problem still to come and it goes by the name of stress.

How so?

Owing more stuff has a deeply repulsive element to it. Last year I happened to catch a scuffle that broke out when greed sweeps the mind and flat-screen TVs go on sale for Black-Friday. It's hard to imagine what kind of TV show would warrant such acts of aggression. And although I offer no proof, I suspect it might have even been the Jerry Springer show … Jerry! Jerry! Jerry! Just sayin', maybe Black-Friday should be renamed Black-Eye-Friday. I digress.

If you do have disposable income, think about buying an experience rather than a thing. My wife likes Chris Stapleton (a musician of sorts) and she recently ordered a ticket to go see him perform live.

The concert ticket was a little more than she wanted to pay, but we justified it because she isn't a typical consumer. Had she paid that much for a new fur coat we might not have seen eye to eye. My point is this, enjoyable experiences are what tightly bond people together. These lasting memories will be around long after all those material things hit the garbage can.

It's really clear that the most precious resource we all have is time. —
Steve Jobs

Given half the chance, kids also seem to get this concept. It's funny how they remember the days when we stopped to color with them on the rug, but quickly forget all the money we spend on plastic toys.

There should be serious economic consequences for any company openly practicing planned obsolescence.

IMPULSE BUYS

Sometimes we are forced to buy things: roofs leak, cars break, kitchens cupboards wear out. I get it. But impulse buys are a totally different animal.

An impulse buy is anything that winds up on your credit card that wasn't a burning desire to buy twelve hours earlier.

I'm not sure who wakes up in the middle of the night and says, "Hey, I must buy another plastic windmill for my garden." It's an impulse buy packaged as a bargain along with a gazillion other bits of junk that we don't need.

The definition of a bargain is something you don't need at a price you find hard to resist.

Buying less clutter (even if it is on sale for $1) inevitably means less plastic heading for the oceans and landfills. If you aren't sure whether something is clutter or not, try to think of it this way: if you don't love it or use it then technically it's become clutter. The two exceptions to this rule are dangly wind chimes and dreamcatchers, even if you love them they are still clutter, — just sayin.

Perhaps when man has exhausted the world's oil supply it will no longer be economically viable to sail plastic cargo all the way from China. It surely adds insult to injury when toxic goods are sold on the open market for one dollar. How is that even a thing?

Sadly, the ones who seem to get sucked into buying those strategically placed "point-of-sale" cheap items are the ones who can least afford to buy them. Bad spending habits are really just that, a habit that stifles cash flow and increases acidic stress. One way to break free is to make a list of all the essential things you need BEFORE you go to the store and then stick to it.

Once self-value comes from owning more stuff it can quickly lead to a never-ending cycle of want. The more we have the more we want. Left unchecked, this line can easily become unhealthy and blurred. If we aren't careful, the things we own begin to own us!

Our perception of success is often judged by the number of dollars we are prepared to exchange for each measured unit of toil. We then exchange a percentage of those dollars for material things. But it's an illusion to think more money automatically equals more happiness.

Okay, what else do we need to know?

Today, more than ever before, the retail industry is keen to help you own more stuff. There's actually a slick psychology in place that constantly manipulates you into buying more things. Gone are the days where the store manager says you are always right. Today, you don't even have to be standing physically inside a store to make a purchase. Now you can shop till you drop while still wearing your PJs. This has the potential to become an alarming problem that goes well beyond recycling. How so?

And here comes the silent killer I mentioned earlier

This is where we come full circle and return to stress affecting our health. As it turns out, your mental and physical health are closely connected to your shopping habits. No really, it's true.

Make no mistake, stress is a killer. According to the American Psychological Association, stress is linked to heart disease, cancer, lung ailments, accidents, cirrhosis of the liver and even suicide!

A preoccupation with accumulating more "stuff" can become a trap that leads to a downward spiral of self-inflicted stress. Somebody somewhere will always seem to have more. And yet this thirst for material things steals the one thing we need more than anything else — our inner peace.

Give a man a million-dollar house and it isn't too long before he's peeking over the garden fence at the sixty-foot boat his neighbor owns. The problem with this concept is twofold.

First- The definition of a boat is nothing more than a hole in the water that must constantly be filled with money.

Second- Ownership is an illusion; we might think we own something, but if that purchase requires any form of maintenance then it can just as easily own us.

> Simplicity is the ultimate sophistication.
> – Leonardo da Vinci

Over the years I've met with some incredibly interesting people. Some of those people were used to seeing more money in a day than many of us will earn in our lifetimes. And yet many were unhappy beyond description.

There's nothing wrong with being wealthy or wanting a better quality of life. But we have to be careful that wanting it (or having it) doesn't take on a life of its own. Many of us have been led to believe that luxury is a standard worth chasing after, yet it also has the potential to bring the most stress.

Throughout this book, I'll always strive to be upfront with you. So to be perfectly honest, there was a time in my own life when I too was a dollar-chasing victim. I followed the herd and drove my pretentious car and even bought the overpriced watch. But no matter how hard I worked it never seemed enough.

Some twenty years later, wealth no longer impresses me. I now find genuine contentment looking at a full woodshed. It brings me comfort to know that I have enough fuel to see me through the coldest of winters. To me, this has a real and tangible value beyond paper money sitting in a bank. Today, I really don't care what car I drive, but I do pay close attention to what food goes on the end of my fork, where things are made, and by whom.

> A man who views the world the same at fifty,
> as he did at twenty has wasted thirty years of his life.
> – Muhammad Ali

If you need help to peel out of a repetitive cycle of buy, buy, and bust then here's an easy three-step way to do it. Step 1: Streamline. Step 2: Use the N-word. Step 3: Repeat.

Step-1: Streamline.

Look around your home and work out which things you really need and which are clutter. How do you know what's clutter? Simple, if you don't use it, or love it then it's not serving a purpose and it's become clutter. (Yup, worth repeating just because.)

Step-2: Now use the N-word.

This is a little trickier because it takes a certain level of practice to say the N-word right. Stay with me on this, it's a great technique and I guarantee it works. Okay, first make an nnnn sound with your tongue (you may need to practice this several times until you feel comfortable.) Only when you have the nnnn sound down can you move on to the next step which is the ohhh sound. Keep alternating between the two sounds and then speed it up a little until finally, a whole new sound evolves into Nnnn-ohhh.

If you are unfamiliar with this sound, it's the opposite of the Yes word. The next time you go shopping trip mentally make this sound when you see the words 50% discount, final reduction, or half off. This one tip alone can help save your sanity, the planet, and your wallet!

STEP 3: Repeat.

From today, continue to use the N-word (NO)when you see the "buy now" button.

NEWS FLASH! Imagine if today, a news flash suddenly came on the radio and said: "Warning you had just fifteen minutes to evacuate your house". What items would you throw in your suitcase? Now ask yourself, what could you leave behind? Hmm, perhaps we don't need as much stuff as we think we do.

What did we learn from this?
Clutter can create self-inflicted stress; the wider implication becomes industrialized pollution and death. Few people are going to stand at our funeral admiring all of those shoes we bought.

Homework: If you are enjoying this book, *please* recommend it to a friend.

Chapter 28

WHEN KETO BECAME KING OVER PALEO

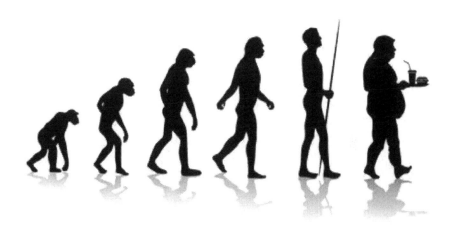

Of all the topics related to health, diet is perhaps the most divided and confusing of all. At times, experts and health gurus will all line up to disagree with each other.

So the aim of this chapter is to bring clarity to the issue and then present you with *six* effective options to keep your health on track. If your diet is currently SAD (Standard American Diet) then any one of the following suggestions is going to be a step in the right direction. That said, it really doesn't matter whether you are currently Vegan, Ketogenic, Vegetarian, or Paleo. **If your health is failing to thrive then something here will be of value to you.**

Every time we eat, we are taking something from the outside world and forcing into our body. The problem is this, the more mainstream a diet becomes, the more we see it backsliding into foods that are trapped inside a box, a can, or a packet. Whenever there is a buck to be made, problems inevitably follow.

Diets come, and diets go, the only thing that matters are, finding something one that works for you. The point I am making is this, good health begins with making good choices. There's actually a freaky correlation between the groceries we keep in our food cupboard and the ones that end up in our belly.

As we now begin moving forward, keeping an open mind will serve you better than becoming entrenched in dietary battlegrounds. The ketogenic diet has been gaining a lot of attention recently so let's explore this diet first.

1. THE KETOGENIC DIET

In 1991 a frozen body was found on a mountain top between Austria and Italy. The ice managed to preserve the body which science estimated was more than 5000 years old! *Why am I telling you this?* To this day, Ötzi's the Iceman" is continuing to reveal how our ancestors lived. Quite remarkably, parts of Ötzi's digestive system remained intact. Any guesses what they found? Yup, a high-fat diet, with moderate protein and vegetables. Today we call this a ketogenic diet. But what does that mean and how do we do it?

Think of your body as a dual fuel burner, pretty much in the same way a hybrid car is capable of running on either gas or electricity. If you eat enough carbs the body runs on glucose. And times when glucose is low, the body is perfectly capable of switching fuels and running on fat.

When the body burns fat, the metabolic state is described as ketosis, but this can only happen when glucose supplies are exhausted. The body then begins to convert fat in the liver into energy cells known as ketones.

In most people, the body has a few days' supply of glucose in the form of glycogen, so the effects of ketosis aren't always immediate. Most people will go into a state of ketosis after several days of consuming less than 20 grams of carbohydrates per day. While this might sound daunting to some, it's worth noting that this process helped your early ancestors evolve. Back then, eating a box full of carbohydrates would have seemed quite odd.

Regardless of whether we find ourselves in times of feast or famine, the brain requires an enormous amount of energy to function. It was once thought that the brain only burned glucose for fuel, but we now know that's not strictly true. Being in a periodic state of ketosis may help to clear the mind.

The full name of what we are describing here is lipolysis/ketosis. Lipolysis simply means that your fat stores are being burned as the primary source of fuel. The by-products of burning fat are ketones, so ketosis is a secondary process of lipolysis. Today people refer to this as a Ketogenic or Keto diet which is really a just shortening of the term.

Once the body enters a state of ketosis it becomes more efficient at burning stored fat. Although the brain is made mostly of fat, it cannot use fat directly for energy, it can, however, use ketones. From time to time I hear the argument that the brain needs glucose to run—and while this may be true, it's actually a very small amount. Interestingly, this small amount can be easily achieved without resorting to eating donuts. How so? Your body is smart enough to make small amounts of glucose through a process called gluconeogenesis.

Essentially what's happening here is we are switching from being a sugar burning mammal into a fat burning one. Some might say this was once our preferred state. Recent studies report that the ketogenic diet can have a marked improvement in diseases such as Alzheimer's, epilepsy, and diabetes. Ketosis reduces blood sugar which in turn reduces insulin levels.

It's worth noting that ketosis and ketoacidosis may sound similar but they are very different. The first, as we have already mentioned, is a metabolic process. But ketoacidosis is a life-threatening illness driven by a lack of insulin. This is typically seen in Type 1 diabetics.

It could be argued that ketoacidosis is a result of consuming more sugar-spiking carbohydrates than the body can process. As I'm sure many of you already know, diabetics produce either too little insulin, or the body doesn't respond to insulin at all. When that happens, blood sugar levels can rise and the blood then becomes dangerously acidic, hence the term, ketoacidosis.

Given that the ketogenic diet strives to lower blood sugar levels, it may be something that some diabetics find useful. As always, before attempting anything new it's best to work with an informed healthcare provider. More so for type 1 diabetics who are dealing with a serious autoimmune condition.

As a final note of caution, keep in mind that although most do fine with the ketogenic diet, a sudden switch to consuming 70% fats may, for some people, be too much, too quick. As always, start small and go slow. Listen to your body for clues which could include pain in the mid- to upper-right section of your abdomen, or pain in the right shoulder. Both are an indication that stress is being placed on the gallbladder.

The Ketogenic diet requires an element of self-discipline. But once you get there, food becomes a matter of choice rather a carbohydrate eating emergency. There's a couple of variations on the Ketogenic diet which include:

• A standard Ketogenic diet which is typically a very low-carb, moderate-protein, and high-fat diet that contains 75% fat, 20% protein, and only 5% carbs.

• A cyclical Ketogenic diet which involves periods of higher-carb intakes, such as 5 Ketogenic days followed by 2 high-carb days.

• A high-protein Ketogenic diet which is similar to a standard Ketogenic diet, but includes more protein with a ratio of 60% fat, 35% protein, and 5% carbs.

On a personal level, I've been in deep ketosis and I liked how it felt. My thoughts were clearer with noticeably fewer food cravings. That said, we are all unique which is why I've taken the time to list five other options below. The first is the caveman diet (aka Paleo diet). It has some similarities to the ketogenic diet as both rely on whole foods.

2. THE CAVEMAN/PALEO DIET

The caveman/paleo diet is a term often used to describe how our ancestors ate long before supermarkets came along and made us sick and lazy. The good news is, on this diet you can eat as much as you like, you just can't eat everything that you like.

This caveman/paleo diet is typically higher in carbohydrates than the ketogenic diet. However, this is a great diet to transition into if you are used to eating lots of processed foods. That said, there's sometimes a tendency to eat more fruit on this diet than perhaps our true paleo ancestors would have. A good way to upgrade the paleo diet is to eat fruit only when it's in season is

3. THE ELIMINATION DIET

As the name suggests, this diet involves cutting out certain "trigger" foods. This isn't a diet to lose weight, it's a diet to lose symptoms. For anyone just starting out, it's worth reminding that the foods most likely to cause a reaction are gluten, dairy, eggs, and nuts, closely followed by corn. Today, it's not uncommon to find all of these foods on one plate!

The trick to the elimination diet is to stack the odds in your favor. This is done by eliminating suspect foods for a minimum of one month. Then slowly reintroduce them into your diet, one at a time. If your symptoms spring back, then bingo, you nailed your problem food.

If you (or someone in your family) are reacting to food, then keeping a detailed food journal is invaluable. Keep in mind that food reactions can happen long after the meal. With so much random "stuff" now added to our food during processing, keeping a written record becomes key.

Once food has become a trigger, simplifying your diet will help highlight problems. If this is a new concept to you, then the elimination diet should be something to consider.

The elimination diet takes effort but the rewards are real. Here's a looong list of symptoms you could potentially be leaving behind.

- Chronic fatigue

- Arthritis

- Asthma

- Mood disorders, including depression and anxiety

- Skin flare-ups like eczema, hives, and acne

- Autoimmune disorders

- Atherosclerosis (hardening of the arteries, a precursor to heart disease)

- Cognitive decline and neurodegenerative diseases, including Parkinson's and dementia

- Learning disabilities like ADHD

- Trouble sleeping or insomnia

- Muscle and joint pain, such as from arthritis

- Weight gain and obesity

- Migraine headaches

- Nutrient deficiencies

- Kidney and gallbladder problems

This isn't a diet you can throw yourself into half-heartedly, and if you aren't mentally prepared to give it 100% then there is no point in doing it.

Why?

When the body reacts negatively to "trigger foods" the immune system makes antibodies to fight the perceived threat. It takes a while for these antibodies to calm down and some believe this process can take three weeks or more. For every nibble you try and sneak, a new bunch of antibodies is relaunched and the whole cycle starts over again. I never said this diet was easy but I am telling you it's going to be worth it. Sometimes we have to give up what we have to get what we want.

Here's what this diet seeks to remove.

- No gluten (or any type of other grain)

- No Dairy

- No Soy

- No refined/added sugar

- No peanuts

- No corn

- No alcohol

- No eggs

That wasn't too bad, was it?

It should come as no surprise that gluten tops the list. Both gluten and dairy have an addictive quality to them, no really it's true. They contain "opioid peptides," yup, that's the same family as opium. Peptides from both gluten and casein (a protein molecule found in dairy) react with opiate receptors in the brain. When a person comes off gluten and casein they can expect to experience withdrawal symptoms.

4. THE AIP DIET

AIP diet stands for Autoimmune-Paleo and it's a leaner version of the basic paleo diet. It also involves the elimination of all the usual suspects such as grains, dairy, eggs, seeds, legumes, as well as some foods found in the nightshade family. Foods in the nightshade family include tomatoes, tomatillos, eggplant, potatoes, goji berries, tobacco, and all types of peppers. The AIP diet is not without merit as it goes a step further and also removes certain trigger foods such as lectins.

5. THE GAPS DIET

Okay, almost there. Four diets down and just two to go. Again, keep in mind that I'm not trying to make your life more difficult. If your health problems have been difficult to figure out, there's a pretty good chance one of these diets will benefit you.

The GAPS diet is another well thought-out diet. Some people claim to have success in treating autism, ADHD, dyslexia, dyspraxia, depression, and even schizophrenia.

The GAPS diet is being mentioned here is because of the dedication of Dr. Natasha Campbell-McBride. I have listened to this lady at length and she has a proven track record of bringing solid results to the table. It also helps that Dr. Natasha Campbell-McBride has not one but two postgraduate degrees: a master of medical sciences in neurology and a master of medical sciences in human nutrition!

The GAPS diet has too many benefits to list, so below is just a small cross-section of the many advantages people often report.

- Psychological improvements

- Boost immunity

- Reduce food sensitivity

- Improve neurological function

- Heal inflammatory bowel disease

- Improve type II diabetes

- Improve lactose digestion

- Kill Candida

- Support detoxification

6. FODMAPS DIET

Our final diet is the FODMAP diet. If you have tried everything else and failed to see a positive result, then welcome to the wonderful world of FODMAPs.

FODMAPs are yet another collection of misunderstood foods that can have a foot in more than one camp. Just as some people are sensitive to gluten, a person with a FODMAP sensitivity will react in much the same way. For some, FODMAPs can be the cause of a wide range of digestive upsets. Particularly prevalent in IBS (Irritable Bowel Syndrome), Crohn's disease, and Celiac disease. And just about any other type of digestive disorder, you can think of.

FODMAPs can be found in a wide range of foods with some foods having a higher count than others. While the list below of FODMAPs is extensive, don't lose heart because I have some good news for you. This condition is unlike a true food allergy and may even be reversible.

A reaction to FODMAPs can be greatly reduced by restricting all FODMAPs for a given period of time to allow the gut to calm down. Are you catching this? I'm saying with a bit of luck; you may be able to slowly reintroduce many of these foods into the diet without too much problem.

If you need more information, then be sure to check out Doctor Sue Shepherd and Doctor Peter Gibson. They recently co-authored a nicely presented book that's sitting at my elbow as I write. As with anyone I choose to recommend, I have no direct link with them other than I admire the work they do. At the moment, very few people are aware of me, my work or my book, so please feel free to mention how you came across their information.

FODMAPS are poorly absorbed by the small intestine and as a result, can enter the colon where they are fermented by bacteria, and as they do so, they draw on water and expand causing excessive bloating and diarrhea.

TEST

There is a standard test that your doctor can carry out that doesn't even require blood to be drawn. It's called the Hydrogen Breath Test and it could save you an awful lot of guesswork.

In case you were wondering, FODMAPs stands for fermentable oligosaccharides, disaccharides, monosaccharides, and polyols. If it's easier, we can simply think of them as fermentable carbohydrates. The list of FODMAPS is extensive so be sure to check them out.

What did we learn from this?
Because there are so many variables, some people may have better success with one diet over another. A little trial and error should set you on the right track.

Homework: If you need the ketogenic diet breaking down a little more check out Dr. Berry on YouTube. Simply copy the link below.

https://www.youtube.com/watch?v=lY87ylWWZYI&feature=youtu.be

Chapter 29

FINDING PEACE IN A STRESSFUL WORLD

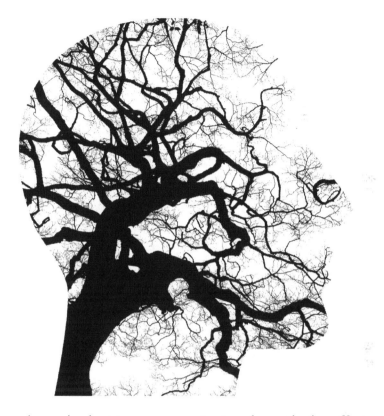

The good news is, short-term exposure to stress has no lasting effects. The solutions that follow are easy to implement and absolutely drenched in common sense.

As for the not so good news, a constant level of stress can manifest itself as headaches, muscle tension, fatigue, stomach upsets, loss of libido, the list goes on and on.

If we crank stress up a gear, it then has the potential to disrupt every system in the body. Immune function decreases, blood pressure rises, and the digestive, reproductive, and nervous systems all become out of balance. Are you getting this bit? It's kinda important.

If left unchecked, stress becomes a silent killer! Rather than try to resolve a mountain of health issues, maybe our time would be better spent today reducing the known causes of our stress.

But first, we should acknowledge that stress affects men and women very differently. Let's kick off with men just because.

MAN-STRESS

Men have the capacity to deal with stress in more extreme ways than their female counterparts. No really, it's true.

Stress can cause a man to become withdrawn, anxious, depressed or display emotional outbursts. I am statistically drawn to the fact that men are also more likely to commit suicide than women. The high-risk group being middle-aged white males. Has stress got your attention yet?

No?

Okay, let's keep going.

When stress gets to this level, it's not one thing but a relentless chain of smaller things that build up over time. It's the constant drip, drip, drip that pushes good men over the edge. To be clear, men who commit suicide aren't always looking to end their lives; they are looking for a way to end their suffering. If this is you, please note that suicide is a permanent solution to a temporary problem.
Men may also have a tendency to internalize things more so than women who (generally speaking) often have a better support network of friends. Perhaps men find it harder to talk openly to their peers for fear of being judged.

So where does a man's stress come from?

The biggest cause of a man's stress can be found in two areas: a need for more money or a need for more time. Essentially, this can mean the same thing. How so?

Men are encouraged to relate success with owning objects, hence just about every automobile billboard is slanted to making a man feel like he needs a high-performance car. This, in turn, requires a man to make more money which then takes up more of his time. Now we are off to the races and we find ourselves in a vicious circle of needing to buy more things. But don't lose hope, the solution coming.

It really doesn't help that men are constantly bombarded with idiotic statements like "Diamonds are a girl's best friend." Or from luxury car manufacturers like Porsche whose catchy slogan claims that "there is no substitute" (for owning a $250,000 car). Really?

If men only knew, ownership is an expensive illusion and inner peace doesn't come from what we buy; it comes from the things we can live without. If we aren't careful, those luxury brands we aspire to own, begin to owns us. Perhaps what men are really saying is they would like to be shown more respect.

TIME

While all men have different income streams, we all get the same amount of allotted time in a day. but what we spend our time doing is a choice. Some men may spend it chasing that latest car, a new suit, or a bigger desk. All of which are rewards for having too much money. But these are short-term rewards that cannot compete with having the freedom to do what we want when we want. Look at it this way.

> A man is a success if he gets up in the morning and gets to
> bed at night, and in between, he does what he wants to do.
> – Bob Dylan

That said, there is nothing wrong with ambition so long as there's a healthy balance. Without balance, a man becomes just another asshole with too many pairs of cufflinks. To be clear, there is no difference between a workaholic and an alcoholic, both must have their daily fix or there's hell to pay. The irony is, few men on their death beds will wish they had spent more time in the office.

LETS GET HIGH

So what's the solution for a chronically stressed man who has fallen into the trap of equating success with ownership of more stuff? That's easy— enrich the life of someone else and expect nothing in return.

Are you getting this bit? It's another important bit.

You can liberate yourself by simply humbling yourself. No really, it's true. There's enough scientific data to support this idea to fill an Olympic sized swimming pool.

The term "Helper's-High" is based on national research done by Allan Luks (feel free to Google). As it turns out, science was able to show that we humans are hardwired to help one another other. Our reward for reducing stress can then be measured both physically and emotionally. Hoorah!

As I'm sure many already know, stress is the body's way of flooding the system with hormones in response to any perceived or real threat. Adrenaline and cortisol pump through the body in preparation for emergency action. Great if there is a Bengal tiger loose in your back garden, but not so great if your boss is a jerk and you are stuck in traffic.

Stress is an omnipresent part of life. But stress that comes from owning more things can be thought of as a being self-inflicted. The fastest way to alleviate this type of stress is to find a problem that's bigger than you are. The good news is this really isn't that difficult to do.

Simply look up from your phone and you will see that people all around you are hurting. Trust me when I say this, to someone who's going through hell, the simplest of human interactions can be more valuable than the shiniest of gold. If you haven't tied this yet, I just know you are going to love how the instant hit of dopamine makes you feel. There is a tangible value to looking a person in the eye and saying, "Hey, are you okay in there, Bud?"

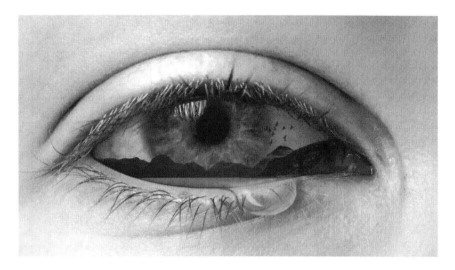

In today's fast-paced world we have become quick to measure ourselves by the quality of the car we drive, the size of our house or the number of electronic digits we have that represent our net worth. Perhaps a man would be better judged not by economic wealth but by the way he treats the most vulnerable members of a society.

Friend, it's not your wallet I'm after; it's you. To those who have the cash to spare, giving money away is relatively painless. Time, on the other hand, has a much deeper value; the love of money gets people into this mess.

Look, I know for some, I'm pushing you out of your comfort zone here. But hear me now, science can show the best way to keep your sanity is to lighten the load of another human being. I'm actually offering you a way out of this shitty cycle, take it!

Man is not made for defeat.
– Ernest Hemingway

This doesn't have to be a drain on your resources, the trick here is to only do a little but do it often. You don't even have to go to a third world to pull this off. Seek and thou shall find as they say. I'd bet the farm (if I had one) that there is someone close to you, either a family member or a neighbor, that's dealing with a form of adversity. What would it take for you to step out of your world and into theirs, albeit briefly?

If I'm right, you will begin to get back something your money cannot buy—a quiet sense of inner peace. No really, have you ever wondered why volunteers don't ask for money? It's not because they have no value, it's because they are priceless!

The idea here is to do what you are comfortable with rather than turning it into a form of resentment. Before you knock on the door of your neighbor you should also be aware that for some folks, the transition into vulnerability isn't always an easy one. Try to be respectful of the fact, people may have lost their financial or physically independence but the desire to have it remains intact.

Do this one thing and a month from now I swear you will be happier and less stressed, you'll also care less about keeping up with the Jones. If anything, the Jones will be looking over YOUR fence thinking, hey, what's with this guy and his new inner peace?

Do this quietly and for the right reasons. Work for a cause, not applause. There's no point if this morphs into a boasting opportunity and no, you don't need to tell the world via a Facebook post what you just did for someone.

NO TIME TO SPARE? REALLY?

If you are fortunate enough to have surplus money in the bank rather than spare time on your hands, then your mission from here is a simple one. *Ready?*

Every year, one million people die from drinking contaminated water. When you stop and think about it, that's a heck of a lot of people with a very basic need that is not being met.

On the flip side, eight men now control as much wealth as the world's poorest 3.6 billion people. According to a new report from Oxfam international, Bill Gates, Warren Buffett, Carlos Slim, Jeff Bezos, Mark Zuckerberg, Amancio Ortega, Larry Ellison, and Michael Bloomberg are collectively worth an eye-watering $426 billion (with a B.)

Don't get me wrong, it's their money, they earned it and good luck to them. But to have an abundance of money parked in a bank, would suggest there's at least a little wiggle room in the budget to help the little guy find water, am I right? So my question to you is this. Why do we expect the superrich to step in and help when we are not prepared to do it ourselves?

As it stands, half of the world's hospital beds are filled with people suffering from a water-related disease? Contaminated water transmits diseases such as diarrhea, cholera, dysentery, typhoid, and polio. And yet, the West continues to send medical supplies to a family dying of thirst. *I digress.*

If you seriously have no time to give, please consider sending a family clean water. A simple google search will show you how.

WOMAN-STRESS

If you think men have it bad, try walking a mile in a woman's shoes— don't get too excited fellas, I didn't mean that literally.

One of the primary causes of stress for a woman is the constant pressure to conform to a certain physical type. Almost every woman who engages with any type of media is immediately faced with images of younger women with increasingly bigger eyes, bigger lips, bigger boobs, and even bigger butts. Sheesh, way to make a person feel uncomfortable in her own skin. If that isn't stressful, I'm not sure what is.

Recently in the U.S., a woman was so desperate for a bigger butt that she turned to an illegal underground practice where bigger butts are offered on the cheap. Sadly, this is done by injecting dangerous chemicals under the skin. These butt-boosting shots include a mineral oil and a can of roadside tire inflator directly into the muscle. Nope, not joking.

If you haven't seen this product before, it's sold in car accessory shops and its intended use is to inflate a blown tire with rapid set expanding foam. What kind of message is being sent out to impressionable young minds that makes them feel the need to pump it up with fix-a-flat tire weld?

Perhaps our wives, sisters, and daughters are being told that they are not enough, and to fit in they need to have a different body shape. If you find yourself caught in this trap I would urge you to seek out an old family photo. Notice how ridiculous fashions come and go? Once it might have been a curly perm, tall platform shoes, or a pair of flared jeans. Now imagine ten years from now looking back at a body that has been surgically altered to meet a current fashion trend?

Given that the global apparel market is currently valued at an eye-watering three trillion dollars, fashions now change before you can say the word overdraft. This can leave some women feeling compelled to buy a new outfit every day of the week!

> Buy less, choose well.
> – Vivienne Westwood

Trying to extract value from ever-changing fashion is just another form of negative stress. Left to ferment, it simply becomes unsustainable as well as stressful. Ladies I beg of you, take comfort from the fact that your uniqueness is your value—it sets you apart from the crowd, so FCUK the fashion industry, and dare to be different!

I get it, we are all longing to be accepted, but in the process, our minds have become polluted with an unsustainable lust for material things. Just as men are striving for more respect from their peers, it seems women, above all else, just want to be valued, but that value needs to come from within.

To add to the problem, social media has now become quick to present us with a carefully staged digital image of perfection. The perfect kitchen, the perfect Christmas tree, the perfect vacation. But scratch below the surface and sometimes we find the deep roots of insecurity.

Perhaps this world doesn't need more skinny women taking selfies in bathroom mirrors. It needs more normal, shaped people doing stuff your Momma used to do. I sometimes wonder if it's called a "selfie" because narcissistic is too difficult a word to spell? I digress.

No matter where we turn, people are desperate to show you an updated snapshot of their happiness. Facebook has become skilled at bombarding us with images of people having fun. But social media can be a warped distortion of reality where nothing much is the way it seems.

Example: I once watched a young mom take at least ten grinning selfies next to a shimmering hotel swimming pool. Standing off to one side was a small child in a damp polka dot bikini complaining that she was cold and hungry.

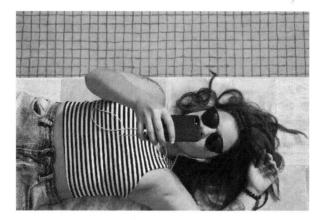

Given the time it took this lady to get the perfect selfie I suspect the kid with the tears in her eye failed to make it to the final cut. Maybe a better name for Facebook would be to call it Fake-book. I guess one advantage of not having a Facebook profile is, you really don't have to worry whether people "like" you or not … just sayin.

What did we learn from this?
Stress can also come from having too little money while trying to own too many things. It can also come from the media, and yes, even social media. We can quickly reduce our stress levels by finding a problem that's bigger than we are, more on this coming.

Stress can also make us more acidic, a subject we seem to keep coming back to. We can reduce our own stress levels by finding a cause bigger than we are.

Homework: Make time to watch this four-minute TED talk by Mark Bezos, this guy is my kind of hero!

https://www.ted.com/talks/mark_bezos_a_life_lesson_from_a_volunteer_firefighter

Chapter 29a

BONUS CHAPTER

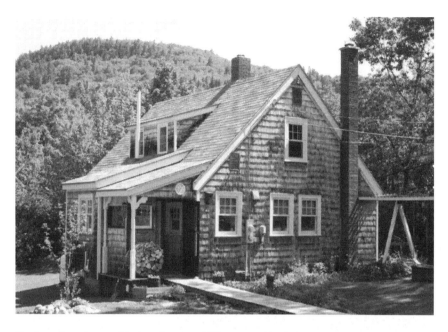

Rather than have this book sound like a medical dictionary, I've tried to keep things interesting by sharing fragments of my own story with you. As I write this, my life is taking an unexpected turn. *Here's why.*

For the past decade, I've been living in the Northern mountains of New Hampshire. It's not a big place or a fancy place, and when we brought this property it needed a lot of work. But over the years we slowly transformed it into a super-efficient homestead.

After my brush with serious illness, home then became an integral part of our lives. It gave my wife and I safe shelter from the outside world; it's our office, church, school and grocery store all rolled into one. In short, we bothered no one and no one bothered us.

Now flourishing on all sides with organic gardens and fruit trees, it's fair to say we have worked every inch of this land. We were intentional about living this way, living simply while growing our own food is important to us. With a small flock of chickens and several sheep, this little gem soon became the absolute epitome of sustainable living.

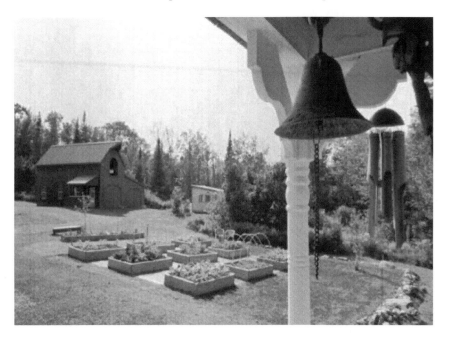

Living this way meant we didn't need a big income. We simply grew what we ate and ate what we grew. Given that our savings had been all but wiped out by illness, this lifestyle fitted us rather well. *Here's where it gets tricky.*

To be clear, growing food year round is hard work, more so when the long Northern winter hits. In an attempt to extend the growing season, I decided to build a high tunnel. This final addition was an important piece of the sustainable puzzle. Little did I know at the time, but this "improvement" was about to be my downfall.

While building the ends of the high tunnel I was careful to make sure they could withstand the strongest winds. I must have built them a little too well because it soon provoked a visit from the local tax inspector.

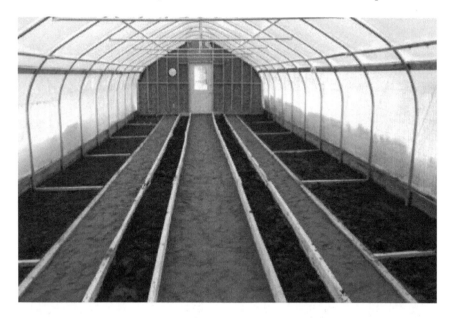

I guess he liked what he saw because he then began sniffing around for a reason to increase our property taxes. The first increase came in at more than $1500. The second increase meant our property taxes had doubled.

When you are trying to live a simple life, this rate of increase was not only unwelcome it was, sadly, unsustainable. Ultimately we were being priced out of our home. The irony is, had we let the place go to ruin, the property taxes would have stayed the same.

With no sign of the man letting up, we knew we couldn't survive another increase. If I'm honest, I'm still a little irritated by this. You know somethings not right when an Englishman gets to complain about American taxation! And so, as I sit and write this first draft, the house went up for sale. Perhaps later we will later see if this if this was a mistake or not.

Either way, a lady from Florida saw the photos online and was immediately smitten. She flew up the very next day and said it was the sharpest looking house she had viewed to date.

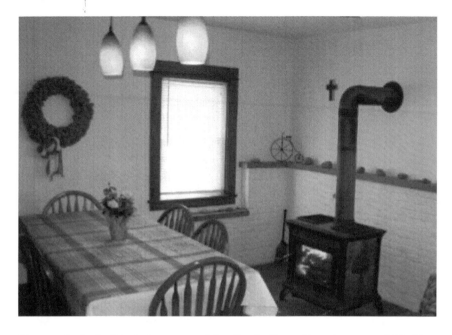

She particularly liked the warm, friendly feeling of our home and kindly commented on how clean everything was. Her husband was suitably impressed with the efficiency of the house which could be heated year-round with just four cords of wood.

This was really important to him (just as it had been to us) because he wanted a manageable place with affordable utility bills. He also liked the barn and marveled at my collection of hand tools all neatly lined up on my workbench like a surgeon's operating table. It seemed to tick all the right boxes, but after several days of deliberating, the wife finally decided not to buy. *The reason?*

She had once traveled to Japan and while there she had bought a large collection of ornamental china vases. For the past fifteen years, wherever she lived, they lived. No matter how hard she tried in her mind, she simply couldn't find a place in our tiny house to put them all. As her husband rolled his eyes for the third time it made me realize this was a classic case of something that they no longer owned. These vases owned them!

Long story short, someone else soon came along and snapped up our homestead. This actually brought heaviness to my soul. My wife and I have fond memories here. But it also made me thankful for the time we had owned this beautiful place.

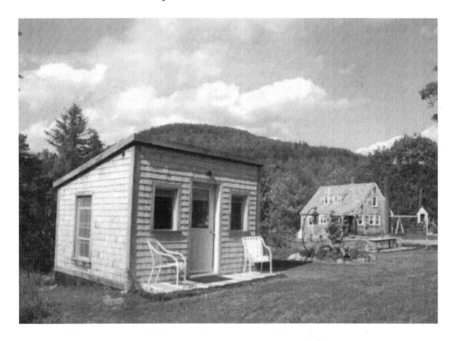

For now, this American dream has come to an end. We have decided to sell everything we own and try our luck back in the motherland. As liberating as this may sound, it's probably the first time I've packed a suitcase and not wanted to be somewhere else.

I'm really not sure where the wind will take us next, and although we will miss the stability of our home, my message to you is clear. Things shouldn't define who we are, because one day, we may have no choice but to let things go

Homework: Look out for the author notes at the end of certain chapters, I'll log our progress here, wish me luck!

Chapter 30

MY DIET IS BIGGER THAN YOUR DIET

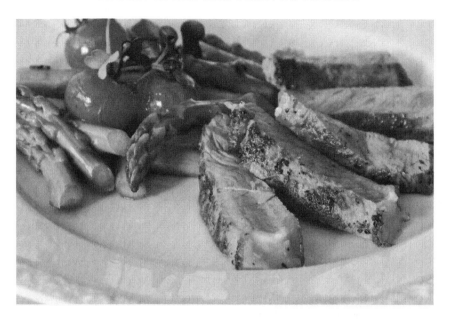

Ask ten foodies what constitutes a healthy diet and you are in for a polarized debate. It seems no topic is more divided than what should go on the end of your fork.

Making a claim to be vegan, paleo, vegetarian, a raw foodist, or ketogenic has almost become like we pledging an allegiance to a particular religion. Rather than divide ourselves into opposing groups, perhaps we can first agree that if your diet improves our health, then it's the right one for you. By contrast, we could say with equal conviction that if you are experiencing health problems, then something you are doing sucks.

When our thinking is rigid it's easy to prove ourselves right, but in the process, we may shoot ourselves in the foot. Once the rigid battle lines are drawn, people are quick to become defensive.

Vegans and vegetarians – I actually respect your point of view. Commercial farming is a barbaric practice at the best of times and I have no beef with you (unintended pun). I hope this book guides people towards those farmers who allow their flocks to be pasture raised.

We could endlessly debate the pros and cons of not eating meat, my goal here is to have readers keep an open mind. Periodically, I find it helps to write down everything I know about nutrition on a blackboard, and then wipe the blackboard clean. What I sometimes find helpful is looking at nutrition from the bodies point of view. More specifically, how does food influence the mitochondria?

MITOCHONDRIA

Mitochondria are tiny cigar-shaped batteries found inside almost every cell in the body. Think of them as the battery in your car. When that battery is fully charged, the engine bursts into life on demand. But when the life of that battery becomes drained the engine is slow to turn over.

Mitochondria really don't care which particular diet group you belong to; they simply demand raw materials to make energy. When mitochondria perform well we feel energized and healthy.
When the mitochondria are undernourished, illness, fatigue, and brain fog are all present. Let's take a closer look at nutrition from the mitochondria's point of view.

ATP

Mitochondria produce energy by utilizing oxygen and breaking down food. They then release that energy in the form of ATP (adenosine triphosphate), along with some byproducts such as carbon dioxide, water, and free radicals. ATP is the fuel of the cell and it's used in everything from blinking to sprinting. ATP is the energy currency of life; its production is more important than the air you breathe.

Think of it this way: you can survive months without food, you can survive days without water, you can survive minutes without air, but when it comes to going without ATP? Meh, you have fifteen seconds or less before you become as dead as a doornail. No really, it's true.

We could think of ATP as gasoline used by a car. As we all know, gasoline doesn't come straight from the ground, it has to be refined from oil. Making ATP is a process and it happens it happens mostly inside the mitochondria. The highest numbers of mitochondria can be found in the brain, eyes, and heart. In females, there are also high concentrations of mitochondria found in the ovaries. Can you see where I am heading with this?

Rather than asking which set of dietary rules we must follow, let's flip the question around and ask, hey, what do my mitochondria need to function optimally? If we know that the greatest number of mitochondria live in our brain which has a naturally high-fat content, then it kinda makes sense to consume foods that are high in (good) fat.

The real kicker is, foods high in good fats are sometimes shunned by the medical profession. For this we can thank a flawed study by the late Dr. Ancel Keys. His work linked higher saturated fat intake to higher rates of heart disease and ever since it seems to have stuck in the minds of some doctors. But the real blame sits with another group of fats known as trans fats. Trans fat = bad. Some research suggests that trans fats can also mess with your insulin receptors.

Trans fats can be found in margarine, vegetable shortening, and partially hydrogenated vegetable oils. And yup, most commercially fried foods are also fried in trans fats. Bad fats won't help your mitochondria; it's the equivalent of trying to build a house with substandard materials. Okay, if we know mitochondria like good fat, it's a pretty safe bet that they also like clean vegetables.

Ideally, aim for six cups or more per day. When buying fresh fruits and vegetables, be aware that some foods absorb more pesticides than others. These are known as the "dirty dozen."

THE DIRTY DOZEN (12 most contaminated foods)

- Peaches

- Apples (always peel)

- Sweet Bell Peppers

- Celery

- Nectarines

- Strawberries

- Cherries

- Pears

- Grapes (imported)

- Spinach

- Lettuce

- Potatoes

12 LEAST CONTAMINATED FOODS

- Onions

- Avocado

- Sweet Corn (Frozen)

- Pineapples

- Mango

- Asparagus

- Sweet Peas (Frozen)

- Papaya

- Kiwi Fruit

- Bananas

- Cabbage

- Broccoli

As a side note, sulfur-rich cruciferous veggies can help the body produce glutathione. These foods would include bok choy, broccoli, cabbage, cauliflower, horseradish, kale, kohlrabi, mustard leaves, radish, turnips, and watercress. There is some debate surrounding the goitrogenic effect of some of these foods which are thought to affect thyroid function. While this may be technically true, it's only in extremely large doses. Cooking and steaming also reduce this effect.

What did we learn from this?

When the mitochondria are fired up they go hand in hand with good health. The eyes, heart, and brain all have a high density of mitochondria.

Homework: For today's homework section I have a real treat for you. Thomas Delauer has a unique gift for explaining things in a way that blends easy to understand videos with the science behind the ketogenic diet. Paperback homies, just go to YouTube and type in the details below.
https://www.youtube.com/watch?v=jpXDQD_5E6k

Author note. As I write this my wife and I are now back in the UK and staying with relatives, at least until we can find a place of our own.

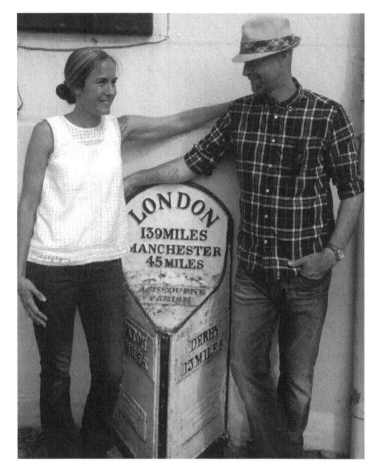

Looking for a new home 2016

Chapter 31

SEVEN BIG GUNS, NO CARROTS

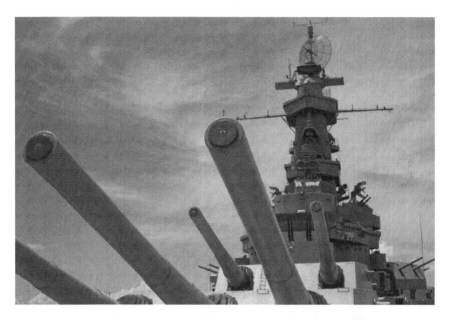

Seven things to improve your health have nothing to do with food. The good news is each is easy to do and totally free!

#1 SET YOUR BODY CLOCK

With the precision of a Swiss clock, birds migrate, flowers open, and roosters crow. Animals, plants, and humans all respond to changes in darkness and light. These changes follow the approximate 24-hour cycle and have a profound effect on physical and mental health. This cycle is also known as the circadian rhythm.

Science recognizes that a "master clock" in the brain coordinates all the other body clocks so that they are in synch. Circadian rhythms influence hormone release, body temperature, sleep-wake cycles, and hundreds of other important bodily functions. Abnormal circadian rhythms have also been associated with diabetes, depression, obesity, bipolar disorder, seasonal affective disorder, etc.

To be clear, the rewards for doing this are rapid and real. Fortunately, resetting your inner clock is pretty easy to do. Within the first few minutes of waking simply exposing your eyes to as much natural sunlight as possible. When our eyes sense morning light, the body responds by being more awake and alert. For that reason, be sure not to obscure the morning sunlight with sunglasses. If you find yourself stuck indoors be sure to turn on lots of bright lights.

If we want to keep our circadian rhythm running on time, it's equally important to develop a regular bedtime schedule. Why?

When the sun goes down we want the opposite of bright light or we risk sabotaging our melatonin production. Keep in mind that before the invention of the electric light bulb humans relied on the soft glow of candlelight. Today we are bombarded with blue light almost around the clock.

> Humans are the only species bright enough to make artificial light and stupid enough to live under it. —Jack Kruse

Blue light also comes to us in the form of laptops, tablets, and cell phones. Be sure to power down tech devices at least two hours before bedtime. You can also apply a filter to them such as F-lux. This is available as a free download and it actually works really well.

#2 MUSIC IS POWER

Music can reach into parts of the brain faster than a shot of tequila. Music has been shown to reach Alzheimer's patients where medications fail. A recent study also showed that music improved cognitive performance and recall abilities in patients suffering from dementia. *No, really it's true.*

Music has the ability to lift the soul. Sometimes we just have to be reminded to use it as part of our daily health routine. For just a moment I'd like to challenge you to imagine living in a world without music.

Now pause for a moment and think of your favorite song. At the end of this article, I'll ask you to play it and see how it stirs up deep emotions. Obviously, the idea here is to lift your spirits so try to steer clear of a sad song.

#3 EARTHING/GROUNDING

Opening ourselves up to new ideas allows us to see problems from a different perspective. You might want to hold onto that thought as we now look at earthing, also known as grounding.

Your brain, heartbeat, and neurotransmitter activity all rely on electrical signals. Without these electrical signals, there would be no life. To be clear, you and I are electrical beings. Grounding allows some of the negative charges from the earth to "ground" our body. We can do this quickly and easily by standing barefoot on grass, stone, sand, dirt or concrete. This experiment will not work on asphalt (that's tarmac for my European homies).

Think about it, apart from that beach vacation, the rest of the year we keep our feet wrapped in plastic boxes. We walk on nylon carpets, drive our cars on rubber tires, and expose ourselves to ridiculously large amounts of electromagnetic pollution.

Now ask yourself, when was the last time you placed your feet on bare earth? For many of us, this probably happens once a year on vacation. Walking barefoot on the beach felt good, am I right?

It's sometimes said, what can't speak can't lie. If we look at blood samples under the microscope the differences between earthed and non-earthed blood are quite remarkable. When the two samples are set side by side it's almost like looking at red wine and tomato ketchup. Yup, earthing improves blood viscosity.

Studies reveal that grounding/earthing has an effect on heart rate variability, cortisol dynamics, sleep, autonomic nervous system (ANS) balance, and reduces the effects of stress. In short, earthing helps put out the fire of inflammation!

Tip—Anytime you find yourself unable to think straight, find a quiet spot and let your bare feet touch the negative charge of the earth. This allows the transfer of electrons to your body which in turn helps neutralize damaging free radicals. In a relatively short space of time, the world and all its problems begin to look like a very different place. Ideally, do this for twenty minutes a day—longer is better, and less is better than nothing.

#4 FIND YOUR IKIGAI

Having a reason to get out of the bed in the morning is probably the most important health tip of all. And yet here it is, tucked away almost undetected. The Japanese have a word for it: it's called ikigai (pronounced ee-kee-guy). Roughly translated, it means having a purpose. It's your reason for being.

Make no mistake—having a project you are passionate about can help keep you out of the doctor's office. It's as if the human soul is hardwired to have a purpose. Trust me on this one, if you want better health, go find your ikigai. When you learn to tap into what motivates you, something happens at the biological level. Ever notice how busy/motivated people rarely get sick?

Every one of us has something we enjoy doing even when there is no money involved. *That* would be your ikiguy!

#5 LAUGHTER IS MEDICINE

It's often said that laughter is the best medicine unless of course, you are laughing for no apparent reason, in which case I suspect you may need some medicine. Laughing in the face of adversity is a powerful cure for all known stress.

Sometimes when my wife and I were waiting at the hospital for my test results, I'd see a worried look come over her face. I'd then find something to make her laugh enough so that no sound would come out and she would be forced to clap like a demented seal. In this midst of adversity, it really was a beautiful sight.

A wonderful thing about true laughter is that it just destroys any kind of system of dividing people—John Cleese.

#6 COLD THERMOGENESIS

WARNING: cold thermogenesis may not be suitable for those with a serious health condition. Please consult a medical doctor before trying it.

Compared to wandering around shoeless with a flower in your hair, cold thermogenesis is a little more hardcore. While it's not for everyone, if you can pull this off the rewards are plentiful.

Cold thermogenesis is a favorite with top sports people to aid in recovery. It can help alleviate pain, improves mood, and increases production of norepinephrine in the brain. It's also known to be helpful in reducing inflammation. But wait, there's more. Cold thermogenesis is said to lower body fat, increase sexual performance, improve adrenal/thyroid function and can even help with migraines.

Cold thermogenesis was something I stumbled upon even before I knew it had a name. Back in 2011 when I was seriously ill my body intuitively knew the value of this, and given how ill I was I just went with it. Years later I was surprised to learn there is actually a lot of published scientific data to support this concept.

Some people find a similar benefit from swimming in the cold sea or sitting in a bath full of cold water. Personally, I've done both of these methods and lived to tell the tale.

You can also start small with this idea by filling a bowl full of water and then placing it inside the freezer. Once frozen, take it out and allow it to sit on the side until it turns to slush. Once you feel up for it, place your face in the ice water for as long as you can stand it. The first couple of times you probably won't be able to do it for more than a few seconds. But over the week you should be able to withstand it for longer periods. Congrats—you are experiencing the benefits of cold thermogenesis with all your clothes on.

#7 LET THERE BE LIGHT

When skin comes into contact with natural sunshine (or light that mimics sunshine) vitamin D is synthesized. The skin acts almost like a solar panel charging up the body with ultraviolet B waves and a cholesterol derivative found in the skin.

Light has an almost magical effect on the body. For those without natural sunshine, artificial light therapy can help to mimic elements of natural sunlight. This form of light therapy affects brain chemicals linked to mood and sleep.

Today, smaller light therapy boxes can fit on a desktop and are designed to help those with a seasonal affective disorder (SAD). This is a form of depression that occurs when sunshine is least available during the winter. Exposure to a lightbox for as little as thirty minutes a day can help stimulate a change in the hormones that affect mood.

RED LIGHT THERAPY

Red light therapy differs from the light therapy just described. Again, it's light that you can see but, as the name suggests, it's a red glow. There are a couple of different types of red light and they each play a different role. In this section, you need to pay attention to those differences because understanding them will impact your health in different ways.

Red light therapy falls into the visible light spectrum between 630–700 nm on the electromagnetic scale. It's often used to treat the surface of the skin. Red light therapy can be thought of as healing and regenerative. It accelerates wound healing and can be applied to muscles or joints to reduce swelling or pain.

I like this option because it's noninvasive and drug-free. There are lots of options out there, some offer good value for the money and others can be quite expensive.

As with any of the following therapies, it's important to keep the light away from your eyes. Ideally, you should invest in a set of inexpensive goggles similar to those used on some tanning beds.

Tip—If you are on a shoestring budget, simply purchase a red heat bulb found in most pet shops. They are sometimes used to keep young chicks warm. If it comes with an inexpensive lamp holder, bingo—you now have red light therapy for less than twenty bucks!

Red light therapy also soothes inflamed tissues, is good for headaches, sinus pain, nasal congestion, sore throats, earaches, and coughing. Red light therapy can help you get a deeper, more restful night's sleep. It promotes relaxation and is believed to reduce anxiety and irritability.

Okay, now here's where we switch to a totally different type of red light so it's important to make the distinction. You should know that the folks at NASA were early proponents of the following types of light.

INFRARED (AND NEAR-INFRARED) THERAPY

Here we are talking about two different lights, the main distinction relates to the wavelengths. Infrared light typically falls into the invisible part of the light spectrum with wavelengths between 700 and 1200 nm, while near-infrared light falls into the spectrum of 700 nm to 2500 nm. Of the two, near-infrared can be thought of as deeper penetrating,

Near-infrared frequency can have a healing effect on our individual cells. Inside the mitochondria (hello again) there are receptors that respond to near-infrared wavelengths. This light triggers an increase in cell metabolism, protein synthesis, and antioxidant activity. This all helps the cells to detoxify. Near-infrared light also reduces inflammation (and pain) while simultaneously triggering growth and regeneration in the cells.

Near-Infrared light comes to us in the form of halogen, laser, and LED. The preferred technology is LED because the surface temperature can be controlled. It also disperses over a greater surface area giving a faster treatment time. Near-infrared LED also has a gentler delivery, will not damage tissue, and carries less risk of accidental eye injury. You can also tap into this technology by joining a local gym that has an infrared sauna as part of its membership.

What did we learn from this?

Each of the light therapies in this chapter offers a wide range of health benefits. Light therapy can affect mood, circadian rhythm, and many other body processes. Red light therapy is helpful with joint and muscle pain and near-infrared therapy can act as a cell rejuvenator, among other things.

Homework: Go play your favorite song as loud as you possibly can!

Then check out Dr. Mercola at mercola.com, or click on this short video below.

https://www.youtube.com/watch?v=2bo_lqFG_20

Author note: It's been several weeks of living out of a suitcase and it's been a challenge to adjust. We miss having our own space and a garden more than we thought possible.

Chapter 32

THE WEAKEST LINK

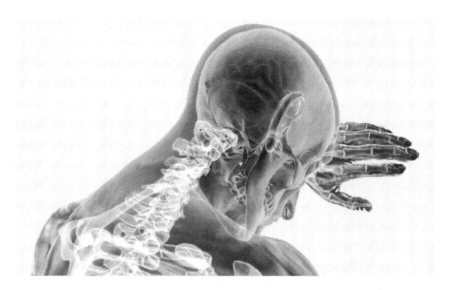

Take a sneaky look behind any website and you will see long lines of computer code. Take a peek behind the dashboard of your car and you will find lots of wires. But if we could take a look behind most chronic illness any clue what we would find?

Yup, chronic inflammation, the two are inextricably intertwined. Wait a second are you catching this? Inflammation is associated with just about every health condition known to man. No really, it's true. PubMed is awash with scientific data connecting inflammation to a long list of diseases ranging from cancer to obesity.

Given the importance of this, perhaps we have things a little twisted. How so?

We have a medical system that's rich in cash and yet it rarely talks about the underlying causes of chronic inflammation. Think about it. In every hospital we have teams of oncologists, cardiologists, and neurologists. But did you ever see an inflammation-ologist?

What's interesting is, developing countries who spend far less on healthcare often outperform the West on everything from infant mortality to longevity. I know, right? What's up with that?

Given the importance of inflammation, let's take a closer look at how it affects the body. First, we should note that inflammation is an essential part of the repair process. Wait a second, did you catch that? Inflammation is a double edged sword, yes it's has the potential to cause problems but it also helps the body to heal!

Problems begin when the root cause of inflammation remains in place. This then allows inflammation to linger longer than the body intended. But what's the difference between acute and chronic inflammation?

Acute inflammation is an early-stage response to obvious physical trauma. Most of us will have experienced acute inflammation (think of a twisted ankle or bruise). Acute inflammation is obvious and rapid. It will include an onset of pain, heat, redness, and swelling. Think of acute inflammation as being a small campfire that's under control.

Chronic inflammation, is less obvious and has more of an insidious quality to it. Think of chronic inflammation as a smoldering, lingering type of fire always on the lookout for a spark. Once chronic inflammation ignites, it can be likened to a raging forest fire.

Chronic inflammation can span weeks, months, or even years. The good news is chronic inflammation is totally reversible. This would also suggest that some illnesses are reversible. If you missed the memo, watch the video at the end of Chapter 5?

Inflammation and illness go hand in hand. All of the steps we have taken to get to this point will help reduce inflammation. From diet to toxicity, it all plays a role. If illness has you in its grip, there is a pretty good chance that something in the below image led to your downfall. If we know that to be true, then by the same token, something here also holds the key to your recovery!

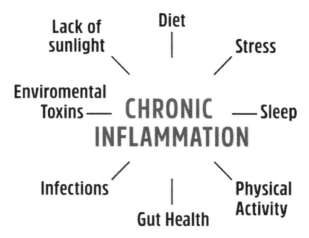

These eight categories can be thought of as our pillars of good health. The good news is once we get these in line, good health is yours for the taking!

If repetition is the mother of all learning, let's quickly take stock of what we have learned so far.

STRESS

Stress has become an omnipresent part of life. Even with the best intentions, it can follow us around like a bad smell. Our jobs can bring us stress, the things we buy can bring us stress, and even the people we surround ourselves with can bring us stress.

> I will not let anyone walk through my mind with their dirty feet.
> – Mahatma Gandhi

Stress can deplete magnesium levels and place a burden on the immune system making us more susceptible to infections. One way to combat stress is to increase the things in your life that bring you pleasure. It's kinda hard to remain in a stressed state when we are doing something that brings us joy.

SLEEP

Some people need more sleep than others but the minimum to recharge is six hours. But the quality of that sleep is just as important as the quantity. Sleep allows the body to carry out internal repairs. Sleep is your bodies maintenance crew that comes in clean up at night.

To get a better night's sleep, be sure to keep your bedroom cool, dark, and quiet. Also avoiding blue light in the evening.

Be mindful of what you eat around bedtime. If you find yourself hungry before bed, try going for a bowl of (sprouted) rice. We aren't trying to win culinary awards here; we are looking for a better night's sleep. Sprouted rice is a slower release of energy compared to less complex carbs.

PHYSICAL ACTIVITY

Motion is lotion for the joints. Cells like movement and even something as simple as bouncing on a small yoga trampoline can have a big impact on our health. If committing to an exercise program is a step too far, then try a brisk walk. Remember, sitting is the new smoking!

When we exercise, our lungs begin pumping more oxygen and this helps with the pH of the body. A subtle way of forcing us to walk more is to park your car away from any stores that you visit.

GUT HEALTH

The gut is the cornerstone of your physical and mental wellness. Feeling grouchy may have more to do with your gut than your brain. Antibiotics can have an adverse reaction to gut bacteria. Restoring gut flora takes time; treat it as a steady marathon and not a fast sprint. Fermented foods and probiotics may prove helpful.

Food plays a key role in both gut health and inflammation. Years of eating the wrong foods cannot be overturned in a day. Here's the scope of the issue. It's estimated that if the GI tract were laid out on the floor, it would fill a tennis court! That's a lot of healing. Bone broths are a valuable tool for anyone looking to repair the gut.

INFECTIONS

Infections are caused by living organisms such as fungi and bacteria. But the key to solving this problem isn't more antibacterial wipes, it's giving the immune system the missing nutrients it needs.

It's often said the number of microbes inside us outnumbers our cells by about ten to one. If that number is accurate then essentially we are a collection of bacteria with a human host. Yup, trillions of bacteria and microbes are already living inside your body. This becomes more of a problem when the immune system is run down or overtaxed.

Most common infections are no match for an immune system that's supported by good nutrition. The problem is we don't always realize this until after we become sick. Bacterial, viral, fungal, and even parasitic infections all receive their nourishment from you. Sugar is their favorite snack.

Natural remedies to help overcome infections may include tea tree oil, colloidal silver, or cistus-incanus tea.

ENVIRONMENTAL TOXINS

All industry is fueled by consumer demand. As long as we buy toxic products they will continue to be made. By 2050, it's estimated that there will be more plastic in the sea than fish! These tiny plastic partials are now entering the food chain and nobody seems to know the long-term effects.

SUNLIGHT

The positive effects of broad-spectrum light on the body are profound. Natural sunlight plays a key role in how we feel, it also affects those tiny energy cells of the body we call mitochondria.

Sensible daily exposure to sunlight also helps our bodies produce vitamin D which is essential for healthy immune function. Sunlight also increases dopamine release in your body. Plants and humans both grow measurably stronger when exposed to sunlight. Light is energy, embrace it!

DIET

As a commodity, food is often exploited; as a medicine, food is often misunderstood. When you buy local food your community thrives and you get to eat food that's in season. Locally grown food has a higher nutritional content than commercially farmed crops.

Fruit was meant to be eaten in moderation and in season due to its high sugar content. Until you get your health issues under control, consider giving fruit the boot. You can slowly reintroduce it into your diet later.

Foods cooked in vegetable oils have been shown to cause oxidative stress. These oils create free radicals in the body which in turn causes inflammation. Oils high in omega-6 will promote inflammation, as will dairy products and grains.

BONUS SECTION

Kidney, Lungs, Skin, and Liver

Treating symptoms is as easy as popping a pill but unless the underlying cause is addressed, progress will always be slow. When we become ill our delicate filtering organs are already working under pressure. Everything we swallow has to be processed by the liver and kidneys. Be aware, anything that comes in pill form can tax these vital organs.

The liver is the most metabolically complex organ in the human body. A healthy liver does far more than just detoxifying toxins. The liver performs over 500 different functions, including fighting off infection, neutralizing toxins, manufacturing proteins and hormones, controlling blood sugar, and helping clot the blood!

The liver plays such an important role that it's the only visceral organ with the remarkable capacity to regenerate itself. Get this: if part of the liver is surgically removed or chemically damaged it can actually regrow itself!

If you find yourself easily crying, becoming easily irritated, or acting out in anger, look to the liver. To help improve liver detoxification naturally, a castor oil pack is sometimes used. The idea is to apply a liberal amount of high-quality castor oil to a piece of cloth, then place it over the liver and hold in place with a hot water bottle to help stimulate lymph and liver function. A simple Google search will give you the exact details for this effective protocol. Drinking fresh lemon juice first thing in the morning may also help improve liver and kidney function.

Gentle herbs such as milk thistle can be helpful to detoxify the liver. Herbs have been used safely for thousands of years, but as with anything that detoxifies – go slow or risk dumping toxins into the bloodstream faster than they can be removed. Using herbs that support the liver and kidneys may help bring an improvement to overall health.

Enlisting the help of a knowledgeable, local herbalist will bring faster, safer results.

As always, do your own research and before trying anything new always speak to your doctor. I sometimes find it helpful to add a small amount of sodium bicarbonate to a glass of water and drink it on an empty stomach. According to research found in the Journal of the American Society of Nephrology, sodium bicarbonate may prove helpful with certain kidney issues.

An indication that the kidneys are running below par is a change in urinary frequency, either too few trips to the bathroom or too many.

These are often reflected in the color of the urine, i.e., too dark or too light. We covered this at the end of Chapter 7.

Once the liver and kidneys are struggling to cope with the demands placed on them you may notice an increase in body odor. With underperforming kidneys, itchy skin conditions such as eczema may also flare up and odor is prominently noticed in the feet.

One reason for increased body odor (and there are many others) could be a low-grade biofilm infection. As mentioned earlier, cistus-incanus tea may prove helpful. When used over a two-week period, most infections give up and the body odor disappears. As always, moderation will serve you better than excess.

What did we learn from this?
It's well documented that chronic inflammation is behind a wide range of diseases. The good news is, something in this chapter might just be your silver bullet.

Homework: for a better understanding of how things link together in the body, check out "How the Body Works," by Dr. John Bergman. https://www.youtube.com/watch?v=nvUuqt94lEE

Author note: Gotta love the British weather. It hasn't stopped raining all week. A black cloud seems to be following us everywhere we go.

Chapter 33

THE 4TH PHASE OF WATER IS LIQUID LIFE

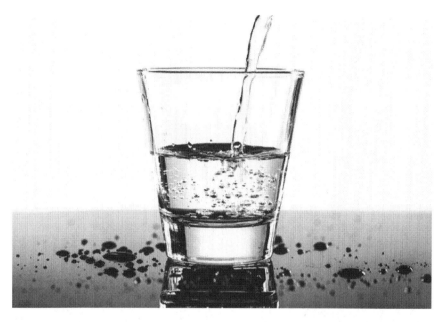

Water can occur in three phases: liquid, solid, or gas. But what if I told you there was a 4th phase to water that's rarely talked about. In terms of benefits to you and your health, this 4th water is capable of tackling a wide range of health problems with astounding results!

When you have this piece of the puzzle in your toolbox it changes everything and, nope, it's not holy water. This is not H20 but rather H302—it's more alkaline, dense, and thicker than regular water. It's actually alive and even holds a negative charge much in the same way that a battery does. To make life possible, this 4th phase water is already inside YOU!

This type of water *isn't* the same as the water we drink from a plastic bottle. This water becomes highly-organized and appears in abundance inside most of your cells, even our extracellular tissues are filled with it.

In this article, we will look at the mind-blowing health benefits of 4th phase water and how to tap into it. First, let's do the basics...

Most medical students learn that water is just a background carrier to more important chemicals and bacteria. But water is central to everything the body does, and in relation, everything the cell does.

Dr. Gerald Pollack, a Ph.D. in biomedical engineering, carried out extensive experiments on this 4th phase of water which uncovered some remarkable findings. One experiment showed that the water molecules acted like telephones to carry messages throughout the body. 4th phase water also has the ability to exclude things it doesn't like, even small molecules. Given this unique property, it's sometimes referred to as "exclusion zone water" or EZ water for short. The negative charge found in EZ water helps form cellular energy.

Are you getting this bit? - It's kinda important.

Your body is made up mostly of EZ water and that water is very much alive! It takes what it needs and excludes what it doesn't. It then sends signals around your body creating enough energy to keep your body moving throughout the day!

A key ingredient for creating EZ water is light (who knew?) whether in the form of visible light, ultraviolet (UV) wavelengths or infrared wavelengths that we are surrounded by all the time. If the goal is to maintain wellness or recover from a serious illness, it's important to understand that energy comes from the light we absorb which in turn affects the cells.

Laser therapy can help increase EZ water by penetrating the cells. In doing so, some laser therapy treatments have also been shown to reduce pain and inflammation which can help shorten healing time in muscles, ligaments, and bones.

Infrared light is the most powerful, particularly at wavelengths of approximately three micrometers. Hence the reason infrared sauna may prove helpful because the cells in the body are deeply penetrated by infrared energy. This, in turn, helps build EZ water. The same can be said for spending time in the sun, although to get the full benefits of natural sunlight you need to step outside rather than sit behind a glass window. Glass will filter out much of the natural light spectrum.

The key here is sensible exposure to sunshine, obviously, we don't want to burn. The fear surrounding natural sunshine and skin cancers is not without justification. That said, it might surprise some to know that when the use of sunblock became more widespread, skin cancer rates failed to go down. What's up with that? Equally confusing is the fact that many skin cancers appear on parts of the body that the sun doesn't reach.

Am I saying you should stay in the sun until your eyeballs burn out? Nope, that would be foolish. But keep in mind some of those sun blocking creams contain toxic chemicals, and anything that goes onto the skin goes into the bloodstream. Who knows, perhaps over time some of those toxic chemicals may prove to be equally problematic.

As we learned earlier, sunshine plays an important role in the way your mitochondria communicate. Increased vitamin D levels also play an important role in creating EZ water.

Personally, I try to get a skin full of sun in the morning before midday. If the afternoon sun is strong I either stay shaded or cover up with a brimmed hat for protection.

Sunlight aside, EZ water can also be found in glacial melt, but unless you have a spare iceberg in the back garden you might want to consider locating a natural deep spring. The deeper the spring the better because EZ water actually increases when under pressure.

There are now products on the market that attempt to emulate this natural process by creating something known as vortexed water. I haven't used any of them myself so I can only speculate about their effectiveness.

Vibration also plays a role in increasing EZ water. Today vibration plates are sold which can be a useful tool to anyone standing or sitting at a desk for long periods of time. If you don't have the spare funds for a vibration plate, a rebounding trampoline also works but to a lesser degree.

EZ water can also be extracted from living foods, which brings us neatly to the subject of juicing. Juicing is simply a way of squeezing the juice out of vegetables and fruits and then drinking the liquid.

If you are unfamiliar with this term you are in for a pleasant surprise. There are few things capable of turbocharging your health faster than juicing!

The good news is, juicing can form part of any diet. This means you can dip your big toe in the water without too much disruption. If you like it, keep going.

Done right, this process will boost your nutrient intake, as well as helping to clean out the GI tract. Over time, this can become clogged with mucus, rancid fats, undigested proteins, and parasites. I know, right? It's nasty, but a cleaner GI tract will result in better absorption of nutrients into the cells. It's often said "you are what you eat" but this isn't strictly true. A more accurate description would be you are what you absorb.

To get the maximum amount of nutrients into the cells, eating large amounts of vegetables every day isn't always sustainable. Even if it were, your poor digestive system would be working overtime to break it all down. Fortunately, juicing allows us to bypass this whole process. This makes those nutrients easier to absorb.

Keep in mind that this is a balance. We don't want to fall into the trap of adding too much fruit. Without wanting to sound like a broken record, once the fiber is removed, fruit becomes a liquid sugar. As always, moderation is key, more so if you are dealing with a low grade fungal or bacterial infection.

WHICH IS BEST?

There are lots of juicers on the market, some big, some small, some are affordable and some can be darn right expensive. Some are quality built and some are junk. Some juicers will outperform others and the tradeoff for doing so can be more time spent cleaning up. So before you rush out and buy a juicer, know that the absolute best juicer to buy is the one you will use. Even a top of the line juicer is useless if it sits in the cupboard because it takes too long to clean.

For sure, buying a juicer can be an investment, but owning a juicer is better than having money in the bank. There are few things in this life worth investing in more than your health—and let's be clear, illness isn't cheap!

Personally, I like the Omega VSJ843. As a first juicer, it's got a decent warranty and it's pretty simple to use. Ideally, I would have liked the excess pulp to be a little dryer, but hey, the tradeoff is that compared to some other juicers it's relatively easy to clean. Before spending your hard earned cash, I would urge you to check out a John who runs a YouTube channel called DiscountJuicers.com. John has an unbiased passion for putting juicers through their paces. If anyone can tell you which juicer will fill your needs, it's John.

Get this right and you can even get the kids to drink their greens! Think apples, with a hint of ginger, mixed with blueberries, celery, and lime, perhaps add a hint of fresh mint, parsley, or even kale. Huh? Relax, kale is nothing more than angry lettuce, and kids won't even taste it.

Before dissing the kale, know that it's loaded with thiamin, riboflavin, folate, iron, magnesium, and phosphorus. It's also a good source of vitamins A, C, K, B6, as well as calcium, potassium, copper, and manganese. Juicing drives nutrients into the digestive system while at the same time packing a nutritional EZ punch. Compared to popping a pill can you see why the health benefits surrounding juicing are unique?

Some people run juicing alongside their current diet, and some use it as a standalone way of intermittent fasting. The trick to juicing is to make your green juice taste good and the good news is there are now hundreds of free juicing blogs to help you.

WHEATGRASS

If we are talking about juicing I need to tip my hat to the subject of wheatgrass. Wheatgrass juice packs a real nutritional punch, and it's something I used to grow when I had my tiny homestead. The vitamins and minerals found in just two ounces of freshly squeezed juice equal three pounds of organic vegetables!

Wheatgrass juice is approximately 70% crude chlorophyll which is nearly identical to the hemoglobin found in red blood cells! Chlorophyll in wheatgrass juice has been shown to increase the function of the heart, help the vascular system, the intestines, and the lungs. It's also said to speed up blood circulation, cleanse the blood of waste, lower high blood pressure, and stimulate healthy tissue cell.

Wheatgrass is rich in vitamin K, which is essential in bone formation. Wheatgrass juice also contains 90 out of 102 vitamins, minerals, and nutrients! I know, right? It beats taking that harsh multi-vitamin.

If you can keep a houseplant alive then growing wheatgrass is totally doable. The grass grows quickly and in seven to ten days will be approximately 8" tall. Then you cut the grass and send it through a hand-cranked juicer. It takes a little more effort, but wheatgrass is another good tool to have under your belt.

Some juice bars now sell wheatgrass but it should ALWAYS be consumed fresh. There's a wonderful book on wheatgrass written by Ann Wigmore. It's a small, well-written book. It's simply called "The wheatgrass book." For me, it's a classic.

MAX GERSON

Finally, while we are still on the topic of juicing, I'd like to give a shout out to the Gerson Therapy. It's a natural treatment that activates the body's extraordinary ability to heal itself. It does this through an organic,

322

plant-based diet, raw juices, coffee enemas (yup you heard me right), and natural supplements. If I had the time to fly to Mexico, I'd make a beeline to the Gerson therapy unit. It has a reputation for helping cancer patients which is why they don't have a base in the US.

If you find yourself in a tight medical spot there is a movie on YouTube called The Beautiful Truth. It covers the Gerson Therapy in more detail.

What did we learn from this?
Nutrients that come in liquid form get to the cells faster while also giving the digestive system a rest. A new juicer can cost as much as a a new Health is an investment, not an expense.

Homework: check out the Gerson Therapy documentary, The Beautiful Truth on YouTube. Here's the link:

https://www.youtube.com/watch?v=jEvQLNg3OJM

Author note: Things haven't quite gone to plan today. The UK immigration system has my American wife jumping through all kinds of hoops. With Christmas right around the corner, they have decided Amanda has to go back to the US and apply for a visa from there. She has a ticket booked for the morning. This will be our first Christmas apart.

Chapter 34

YOU HAVE A GIFT

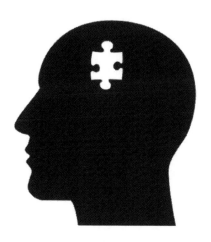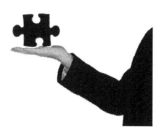

In this life it pays to know and who you are. To help you find this out you have no choice but to embrace where you came from. Me? I grew up in government housing. It's a part of me, and for better or worse, it has shaped and molded my unique personality.

Back then, life wasn't always perfect *but it was always interesting.* At times, people were quick to settle their differences the old fashioned way, standing toe to toe with clenched fists. Thus ensuring the ointment of life always had an element of grit to it. If you allowed it to be, it could be an intimidating place to live. But in the middle of this madness, I was fortunate to have someone in my corner who was respected by all.

Dad was one of those unusual people who could turn his hand to anything and do it well. He could fix the toaster and play the guitar; he even knew his way around a boxing ring. With his magical tricks and witty jokes, he could entertain a room full of people with ease.

At the age of fifty, he suddenly started running in marathons and, just for good measure, he always crossed the finish line by doing a forward roll –

in spite of his bad back. He once grew a prize vegetable garden from seed, he then rewired the whole house to an impeccably high standard!

A meticulous maker of intricate things; he lived his life free of debt and spent money wisely. He never drank and he never swore. Over the years he also developed an uncanny knack for being right and people often came to ask his advice.

And yes, he could fix the TV set and the car, but Dad's greatest gift was his writing. His beautiful handwritten notes always carried a beautiful majestic flow. Writing seemed to light a fire deep inside him. In his spare time, he would leave notes for anybody who would read them. Before leaving for work he often left Mom a page-long letter, and when eBay first came along he spent an hour writing the most eloquent description just to sell an old coat. It's fair to say Dad's writing was not only his gift, it was his passion. The problem was he didn't know it, and so he settled for less.

For most of his working life, he fed his family by driving a big red, double-decker bus which due to his precise nature, always ran on time. His bus driver uniform was always neatly pressed in a certain way, and his clean, polished shoes stood out from a meter away.

Dad never skipped a day of work, not even when he was ill. With an unblemished driving record that stretched more than three decades, his number one goal was to deliver people safely to their destination. It's fair to say he was honest and friendly with everyone he met.

Late one night a man boarded and left his wallet behind. The next morning the wallet found its way back to its rightful owner. Another night a drunk got on the bus and spat in dads face – he wasn't quite as easy to trace. If you asked my dad why he drove a big red bus he would always joke, "It's an easy job, my load walks on and walks off." He tried to find a positive in every situation. Dad was gifted in so many ways and I'll never know why such a meticulous mind spent ten hours a day driving a big red bus.

It pains me to say it now, but dad wrote me so many eloquent handwritten letters that I'd sometimes catch myself skimming through them. If only I'd known back then I would have said, "Hey Dad, why don't you write down all those practical tips that you know?"

He often told us things like, "Never buy a house at the bottom of the hill."

Earlier this week the local news ran a story about a street that had been flooded out, except of course for the one house that stood at the top of the hill. Sadly, my dad's not here anymore so my question to you is this. What's your passion and why aren't you doing it? In this chapter, we will find out.

WHO ARE YOU?

To better understand ourselves it's important to understand who we are. Are you introverted or extroverted? Do you lead with your head or your heart? Are you goal oriented or people orientated?

There are 16 different personality types, but do you know which one you are? To help you find out please see the below link. It's a completely free test and you may find it's a little freaky how accurate it is.

TEST

https://www.16personalities.com/free-personality-test

JUNG

Swiss psychiatrist and psychoanalyst Carl Jung founded analytical psychology. He believed our distinguishing characteristics have a tendency to fit into four basic personality types. For ease of understanding, Jung color-coded these four categories using the colors yellow, red, blue, and green. See if you can recognize yourself in any of them. *Ready?*

YELLOW

Yellows like to be around people and are very much the life and soul of the party. They are sociable, expressive, imaginative, and enthusiastic. They are also informal, optimistic, and animated. Yellows have creative imaginations that can sometimes run away with them as they are very fast-paced thinkers. Yellows don't like to be slowed down with intricate details or formalities.

RED

Reds like to take control. They are strong-willed, fast-paced thinkers. They are risk takers, purposeful, less patient, overtly competitive, formal, and rational. They don't like small talk and prefer people get straight to the point. Hence, I've left this description short just for them.

BLUE

Cool blues are deep thinkers, analytical in nature, very detail focused and formal in their thinking. They are deliberate, systematic, precise, and pay great attention to detail. They like things in their place and have excellent time management skills. They are much slower paced than the reds or yellows. Blues like to have all the facts and then logically put together a suitable answer. Blues don't like to be rushed into things or be disorganized.

GREEN

Greens are laid back, relaxed, and patient. They are easy to get along with and informal in their approach. They are social and focus more on relationships and may at times come across as emotional. They are much slower paced in their thinking and are very democratic people. They are very understanding and agreeable. Greens sometimes make the perfect go-between for Reds and Yellows, who are much faster paced. They also act as the facilitator to conflicts. Greens don't like to be pushed or put on the spot.

Did you see yourself in any of these four groups? How about family members or your partner? As for me, I'm probably 85% blue and 15% red.

Knowing which color best suits your partner can help unlock those complicated interpersonal relations. When we choose a partner we are sometimes drawn to personality types that are opposite us. We can then spend our whole lives being driven crazy by them, and they us!

If you want to show your affection to a green, give them a hug, if you want to show affection to a red, offer to complete a task in record time, lol. Knowing what makes another person tick is halfway to a lasting relationship.

Just as important, is when we understanding our own role in the workplace. When we are happy in our work we are naturally less stressed. All too often we base our entire working lives on our academic achievements. This, in turn, the has the potential to becomes an endless source of inner friction. I sometimes wonder why careers advisors aren't trained to pay more attention to specific personality traits.

If you are currently stuck in a job that you dislike this chapter may prove particularly insightful. The good news is it's never too late to change. The privilege of a lifetime is being who you are – Joseph Campbell.

When you look at the diagram below there are no right or wrong answers, only relevant ones. Check which category best suits your personality best and then see how it could be put to good use in a working environment.

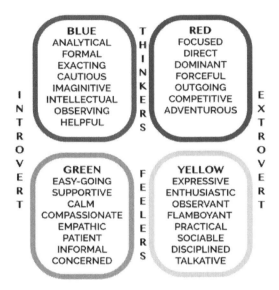

If we relate these colors back to the workplace, can you see a blue introvert working in customer sales? Nah, I don't think so. How about a yellow extrovert working in sales? Hmm, maybe. How about a fiery red dentist? Nah, I think I'll take my chances with the more supportive green one. My point is this: the only way to do great work is to love what you do. If you hate your job, it's gonna show in your work.

FIND YOUR GIFT

No matter which color you identify with, you, my friend, have a gift buried somewhere deep inside you. A clue might be that subject that you love to talk about. Once you know where to look, your gift is actually pretty easy to find. What's the one thing that seems easy or obvious to you, while others may struggle or muddle their way through? Congrats, that would be your gift.

> The meaning of life is to find your gift;
> the purpose of life is to give it away.
> – Picasso

Once you have your gift, own it, nurture it, **fight for it.** It's the only way to a meaningful life. All too often we are told we must run with the pack, swim with the current, or follow the crowd.

With bills to pay life is very good at getting us to comply. But when we obey the rules we accept the limitations imposed by others. If we aren't careful we become conditioned to think it's too late to change. Perhaps this was the reason my Dad drove a big red bus for most of his working life.

From time to time you may hear well-meaning phrases such as "Do what you love and all good things will come". This should be easy to do right? *Meh, not so fast.*

Let's not forget that some of us were educated in decaying inner city schools and taught from an early age to think *inside* the box. – such impressionable young minds all programmed to expect and accept less.

I don't ever recall my teachers every saying, "Follow your dream, do what you love, we believe in you!" Instead, we were told to face the wall as a punishment for not being able to recall information on demand. For someone like myself who suffers from a form of dyscalculia, this technique did more to suppress the human spirit than teach the basics of math.

It's fair to say my substandard education has made writing this book more of a challenge. Yes, I have my voice, and yes, I have a message that I am keen to convey. But none of this came easy.

SO WHO IS JAMES?

From the first page to the last, I've always been open and honest with you. So yes, it's true. I'm *not* a professional writer, I'm just a guy who dared to dream of one day becoming one.

I guess I've always been a square peg in a round hole. **Or perhaps because I'm *not* a part of the medical establishment I'm able to see things from a totally different perspective.** My goal has always been to cut through medical BS and present otherwise dull topics in a way that become interesting to read. This is my true passion in life and I hope I'm doing it justice for you.

But like my dad before me, I spend most of my time doing work that perhaps I'm not destined to do. As I've been writing this book it might surprise you to know that I've been paying my rent the only way I know how to, the hard way – with my hands.

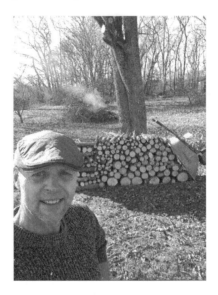

Yeah, that's right, shock horror, I'm a real person. The one without a *without* a college degree that you call to clean up your yard or fix that broken window. You see, **I'm still fighting for my gift** and for the moment, the world doesn't care that I have the ability to simplify complex topics and make them enjoyable to read. But I'm determined not to let my substandard education define who I am so in the winter months, when work is thin on the ground, I read.

The capacity to learn is a gift; The ability to learn is a skill; The willingness to learn is a choice. – Brian Herbert

Whenever I'm asked the dreaded question of what I do for work, I cannot claim to be a writer, although this is how I've been spending my evenings. So I usually reply, "I just fix stuff." This is generally met with a silent nod.

Ever wonder why people like to pigeonhole us like this? It's their way of calculating how much respect to give a person. I'm currently toying with the idea of telling people I blow up bridges just to gauge their reaction, lol.

Attempting to balance physically demanding work, and write an epic health book, *and* find a new home has been a challenge. With hindsight maybe this year wasn't the best time to try and write a new book. But **when something is important to us we either find a way or we find an excuse,** and nobody cares how good the excuses are for *not* doing something.

During my own illness, I quickly found that when you are the one sitting in a wheelchair it doesn't matter what the certificate on the wall says. The only thing that matters is if the solution works or not. Here's an example of that.

BROKEN TOILETS AND KNEES

Recently, while carrying out some basic home repairs for an elderly homeowner I also noticed he had a problem with his knee. As a general rule, I try to keep my thoughts to myself for fear of being misunderstood but the poor fella seemed to be in obvious pain.

To fix his broken toilet, I replaced the inlet valve, to fix his knee I suggested he apply dimethyl-sulfoxide (DMSO) directly to the area twice a day and then refrain from eating all reactive foods in the nightshade family for one month. From the look on his face, I guess he thought handymen only fixed toilets.

Fortunately, he was in enough pain to see past my stained overalls and within a week the treatment had taken most of the inflammation out of the joint. The customer was grateful even if he was a little mystified as to why he could suddenly walk unaided. Sometimes it feels as if I am drawn to people with unusual health problems although it doesn't always pay to speak up.

I once installed a kitchen cupboard for a lady whom I overheard complaining of eye pain. When I suggested she should immediately get herself checked out by a doctor, she scoffed at my advice. I know, right, what could the handyman possibly know about optic neuritis? A week later she called me to say that her doctor had confirmed the very same thing. Although I suspect he charged her a little more than I was getting for the repair work.

So by now you are probably now wondering how does a fifty-something, often underemployed handyman come to know all this stuff? Well ... if you were paying close attention you will already know from Chapter 2 that unbending persistence requires no skill, it's nothing more than the noble art of being knocked down ten times and getting up eleven. The trick is to bring it out in the open where it can be of most use to us.

Is it easy? No, here's why ...

Whenever I pick up my tool belt my wife knows we can expect to get a paycheck on Friday, when I pick up my laptop I sometimes hear this uneasy loop playing over in my mind – "Give up, stick to what you know, you will never be a writer, you are letting everyone down, yadda, yadda, yadda.

In my darkest hour when I was on the verge of giving up on my dream of becoming a successful writer, hope came from my daughter. Her simple note that follows has been driving me to see this project through to the end.

Dad-

I want to remind you of something. You're not writing this book for you, you are writing this book for people who have little hope left, for people as ill as you were, who have no way to get out. You're writing this book for your kids and your kids' kids. You're writing this book because you said you wanted to help people. You wanted to write this book so that nobody had to go through what you went through.

You are writing this book for a reason, for a purpose. You were meant to be a writer, not a carpenter, not a mechanic, not a handyman. You were meant to mean something, to change something, to be an inspiration to people who have none left. There's a fire inside you to write, a certain creativity. You were meant to be a writer and I just wanted to tell you that.

P.S. I Love you. X

It seems that regardless of my current situation, this book isn't going to leave me alone until it's finished and I have no business quitting.

What did we learn from this?

We are conditioned to believe our dreams are foolish. Find your gift and then use it to do what you were put here to do.

Homework: you can see Dr. Jacobs talk about the healing power of DMSO (Dimethyl sulfoxide) for yourself by watching the short video clip below. Keep in mind there is no big money to be made from DMSO which is perhaps why some people like to jump all over it.

DMSO is sometimes used to help protect delicate donor organs while they are in on their way to transplant patients. The FDA also approved DMSO for the treatment of interstitial cystitis suggesting it has a valid place in medicine. Am I saying DMOS is right for everyone? Nope, never did say that, but for someone facing the surgeon's scalpel and a 50k bill for a knee operation, it pays to have a few options on the table.

The DMSO video clip below is taken from 60 minutes and although it's a little dated, the information remains as valid as ever.
https://www.youtube.com/watch?v=H_szhaOS9V4

Author note: Okay so it's been about a month or so since my wife Amanda returned to the US. Rather than get ourselves bogged down in more bureaucratic British red tape, we have decided it would be easier if I also returned to the US.

Chapter 35

FALLING DOWN

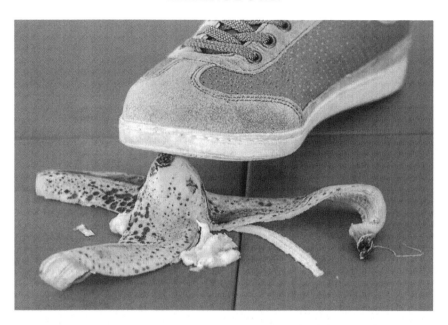

While I haven't always been a country boy, it's fair to say I've always been a homeboy. Recently, the adventure of looking for a new home has worn thin. The uncertainty and upheaval has brought a heaviness to my soul. I miss my orderly life, my OCD vegetable garden, and a familiar place to hang my hat.

Living in a state of limbo is stressful. We now find ourselves back in the US and living in a rented apartment. It's fair to say this has been something of an adjustment. But compared to another day of living out of a suitcase we are, for the moment, learning to embrace our new environment.

Being out of my comfort zone will no doubt come through in these final few chapters. Perhaps it wasn't the ideal time to try and write this book. Perhaps it's refreshing to learn that there are days when we all struggle. Even at the best of times, this path to clean living isn't always easy and the best-laid plans can easily misfire on us. As John Lennon once said, "Life is what happens while you are busy making other plans," although he also said, "I am the egg-man, I am the walrus." Sadly, John is no longer with us so we can only guess what he was smoking at the time. I digress.

As mentioned earlier, I've spent much of the past decade living in a small rural community growing my own food. I'd also gotten to know all the local farmers by name and even had access to a local freshwater stream. Today, things are a little different. The tranquility of listening to a babbling brook has been replaced with whoever lives upstairs walking across my ceiling.

As I learn to adjust back into city life, I've suddenly taken to sucking water out of plastic bottles. It's not that I'm being lazy when we sold our tiny homestead in Lancaster NH it made no economic sense to ship everything to the UK.

Being disconnected from all the things I had come to rely on has shown me how difficult it is to maintain a healthy lifestyle on the fly. So I'm afraid you are going to have to tolerate a little more of my disappointing honesty. I'm a real person and sometimes I mess up. This past week my once pristine diet has also fallen.

I'm not going to explain why it was in the cupboard, but in a moment of weakness, I ate a whole stupid box of wheat crackers. *I know, right? What's next, Flakka?*

I accept that most health gurus rarely put a nutritional foot wrong as they are carried from podcast to podcast on the shoulders of infidels. Alas, I can no longer claim to have the same high standards.

As stressful as things are at the moment, it's also inspired me to write these remaining few chapters with fresh eyes. I've now come to realize that without access to a private chef, there is going to come a time when we find ourselves standing in a sterile supermarket feeling overwhelmed by it all, am I right?

Take comfort my friend, know that we are not the first nor will we be the last to fall off the gluten wagon. There is no point in beating ourselves up over it; tomorrow is another day and we must pick ourselves up, dust ourselves off, and go again. If this is you, take a deep breath then draw a line under today and begin moving forward. Whenever I fall from nutritional grace, I find it helpful to ask: why the hell am I doing this, anyway?

Maybe, like me, you are just sick of being sick. Maybe you are simply tired of being tired. The only right answer is an answer that motivates you. Finding something that motivates you is pretty important. – fear, pain, accountability, and family are all powerful motivators. Knowing which one motivates you can make the difference between success and failure.

As for me, I'm making myself accountable. Over the next few chapters, I'm going to challenge myself to give you the healthiest options I can find. All while living on a tight budget and with very little time to cook. To make things more interesting, I now have a concrete slab for a garden and a landlord breathing down my neck.

What I'm about to suggest isn't going to win any culinary awards, but the idea here is to say hey, I get it. Not everyone has the time or money to find organic food grown by a one-armed monk. This is do or die, and the "do" part sounds better than death. Let's see how this pans out, you in?

What did we learn from this?
We all mess up – own it. Quit whining about it and try again.

Homework: Check out this short video by Kimberly Snyder, here she offers simple advice for those looking to find a healthy pizza. If you get the opportunity, please feel free to mention where you found her information.

https://www.facebook.com/KimberlySnyderCN/videos/1510961885593465/

Chapter 36

WHAT THE HELL DO I EAT FOR BREAKFAST?

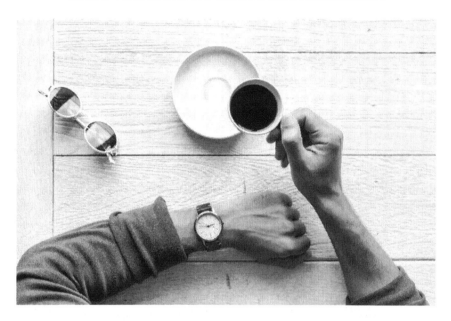

It's often said that breakfast is the most important meal of the day, this is the one piece of mainstream advice I think we can all agree on. Alas, not for the reasons you may be thinking. Breakfast is the most important meal because getting this wrong can set up failure for the rest of the day.

Starting the day off with a boxed cereal containing dried fruit, grains, and added sugar is a sure way to promote inflammation. Add a splash of cow's milk and we now have a cereal killer on our hands.

Now we know what breakfast isn't, let's be clear about what breakfast is. Breakfast literally means, "breaking the fast" and it's usually the first meal we eat after sleeping. For some of us, it could have been twelve plus hours since our last meal, although this isn't necessarily a bad thing. *Here's why.*

Given that the average breakfast choices are cereal, toast, or fruit we might be better off eating no breakfast at all. Hear me out and this becomes intermittent fasting is something I do often and it ties in nicely with the ketogenic diet. When we push back on the morning urge to eat sugary carbs two things happen: first, we aren't being slowed down by excess sugars. And second, the body is encouraged to burn more fat in the form of ketones.

I know our time is short so I'll resist the temptation to write a whole chapter on IF (intermittent fasting). Just know that it's a process that actually dates back to biblical times and the science behind it is pretty impressive.

Either way, in this chapter I've set out seven simple breakfast ideas to help you break away from all those sugary carbs. All of these ideas are quick to make and require very few ingredients. Best of all there are no calories to count. The idea here is to give you a few *workable* meals as opposed to being a culinary tour de force.

BREAKFAST IDEA #1, THE BULLET

Up until now, I've been pretty good at taking things away from you and your reward for sticking with me is about to be repaid. How would you like a breakfast that gently lifts brain fog and gives you more energy? This breakfast idea will make you feel good and, in the process, you won't even feel hungry until mid-afternoon. Welcome to the world of butter-coffee!

Butter coffee is the brainchild of Dave Asprey. Dave is one of those curious people who like me refuses to accept illness as an acceptable destination. And while he makes no claims to have invented intermittent fasting, he certainly came up with a better way to do it.

Whenever I read a study relating to coffee, the quality of that coffee is rarely taken into account. This is huge because the difference between regular coffee and high-quality coffee is night and day. When the two are treated the same, results are always going to be skewed. To be clear,

Bulletproof coffee is an upgraded version of the stuff sold in your average coffee shop.

Ever wonder why your cup of Joe makes you feel good and then a few hours later you crash? It's all to do with where and how and where the beans were harvested. Once mold gets into the coffee harvesting process it produces a toxic chemical known as a mycotoxin.

Beans grown at higher elevations are less likely to be affected by molds. For that reason, it's best to stay away from blends that often include beans from lower down on the mountain. There are lots of high elevation coffee bean producers out there and Dave also has his own brand. Bulletproof coffee is a little pricey but I'm assured it's carefully screened for molds. If you try Dave's coffee, be sure to check out "The Mentalist."

Coffee sometimes gets a bad rap for stressing the adrenal glands. This is something I am well aware of, but let's not be in a rush to throw the baby out with the bathwater. If you are suffering from any type of adrenal dysfunction, supplementing with cordyceps has a wide range of health benefits. Cordyceps have adaptogenic properties which is something we will look into later.

Butter coffee can be used as an alternative to eating those energy-zapping cereals for breakfast. Butter coffee is easy to make, but in order to pull it off, you only need three key ingredients.

1. A high-quality coffee bean from the higher elevations.

2. MCT oil which is a form of saturated fatty acid.

3. Grass-fed butter such as Kerrygold.

Note: Inferior substitutions will not work.

A deeper reference to these key ingredients can be found just below by clicking link.

Dave can also be found on his podcast Bulletproof radio which I tune into often. I would have liked to send Dave a copy of this book. Unfortunately, I wasn't able to find a direct mailing address form him. *If you get the chance to speak to him, would you please make him aware of this book?*

See how-to make Bulletproof coffee below

https://www.youtube.com/watch?v=4YjLMdx3YZY

BREAKFAST IDEA #2, BACON SALAD

So in true ketogenic fashion, our mornings look to be leaning toward the higher fat and lower carb spectrum. This leads us neatly into the super easy bacon salad.

I'll award bonus points if you can get your salad from the local farmer's market, but if you are in a bind simply pick up a box of mixed salad from the store.

These types of pre-made salads aren't perfect, but they are a gazillion times better than toast for breakfast. I'll even give you bonus points if it's organic. If not, don't panic, just do the best you can.

I'm not going to micro-manage you on the bacon, you know how you like your bacon cooked better than I do. So long as you aren't cooking it with bad fats then you have a green light. While the bacon is cooking grab a clean plate and throw a handful of mixed salad onto it. Add a squirt of apple cider vinegar and a pinch of Himalayan salt. As soon as the bacon is done, add it to the salad eat. The simplicity of this meal means food triggers are kept to a minimum. If you have it in the cupboard, adding a little olive oil will help get the fat ratio up, as will MCT oil. At a stretch, you could also melt a little Kerrygold butter over the bacon.

You might be wondering why eggs are missing from the bacon salad. While it may be true that eggs are nutritious, some people react to them.

For now, let's try this breakfast without the eggs and then a week or so down the road try adding them in and see how you feel. Remember, some trigger food reactions can be delayed and subtle, such as general fatigue.

BREAKFAST IDEA #3, GO-AVOCADO

Technically avocados are a fruit but they have a lot of vegetable-type qualities. Avocados are nutritionally dense and a better source of potassium than bananas. Do I like avocado? No, I can't stand the damned things but it's another form of good fat and if it keeps me on my feet then I'll eat them. What I do like about Avocados is they are a super "fast-food". Once cut it half they will stave off hunger for the next few hours.

Although the idea is to limit fruit for breakfast, adding a little lime juice and a few blueberries makes an avocado more palatable. You can also add a pinch of Himalayan sea salt for another bonus point. Avocados come loaded with heart-healthy monounsaturated fatty acids. Need more fiber? Go avocado.

BREAKFAST IDEA #4, BUDWIG

If aren't sensitive to dairy, the Budwig breakfast could be an interesting fit. This idea is accredited to German biochemist Johanna Budwig, a highly respected pharmacist. She held degrees in physics and chemistry and was nominated seven times for the Nobel Peace Prize. Johanna Budwig lived to be ninety-five and was obviously a very smart lady. Her simple Budwig diet has been suggested by some to be a powerful protocol for certain cancers. Am I saying this is a cure for cancer? Nope, never did say that, and never would. I just thought you might find it interesting. You can find more information relating to this on a website called "The Cancer Tutor".

The reason I've included the Budwig breakfast here because it's simple to make, it tastes good, it's fast and the ingredients are minimal. For this we need organic flaxseed oil and some organic cottage cheese (or sheep's milk quark if you can find it). You can also add a few berries if they are in season.

Here's how you make it:

Place 6 tablespoons of organic cottage cheese in a mixing bowl.

Add 3 tablespoons quality flaxseed oil. Note: only buy flaxseed oil from a store that keeps it fresh in a refrigerator and always check the sell-by date.

Add 2 tablespoons freshly ground flaxseeds

Whisk it all together with a simple immersion hand blender and you are good to go.

Optional: if you want to make it more palatable, throw in a handful of berries or ground nuts.

BREAKFAST IDEA #5, OKAY-OATS

There are times on the ketogenic diet when you may need to refuel with a few carbs. Buying plain oats ensures you aren't subjecting your digestive system to added sugars. You can make plain oats more interesting by adding nuts, berries, or a shake of cinnamon. It's important to steer away from mass-produced oats as they are almost certainly cross-contaminated with gluten during processing.

Oats are quick to make and a good source of fiber, simply add hot water. Don't waste your time buying instant oats which almost certainly come loaded with added sugar. Instead, soak plain oats in a bowl of water overnight. In the morning simply strain them and heat them in a saucepan with a little fresh water or almond milk. Viola! They are as fast as instant oats without all the additives.

BREAKFAST IDEA # 6, MINI-MASTER

Some mornings you might not feel up to eating a big breakfast, and that's okay too. If this is you, simply make a mini master cleanse. This drink will not only help to detoxify your liver and kidneys it can also keep hunger at bay for a few hours. I find this works best with room temperature water.

Add the juice from one freshly squeezed lemon to twelve ounces of water. A mason jar works great as the measurements are on the side of the glass.

Mix in a pinch of cayenne pepper, shake and drink. If you aren't too worried about being in ketosis a teaspoon (or less) of pure, dark maple syrup. This combo is part of the Master-Cleanse and I sometimes use it to replace breakfast. Don't be afraid to mix this up a little. I usually do this without the maple syrup and I'm still here to tell the tale.

BREAKFAST IDEA # 7 HEALTHY ALFIE

You aren't the only one who likes to eat breakfast, so do your gut bacteria (hello again). Some of them like to feed on pre-biotics which come in the form of fiber. Given that the ketogenic diet is essentially low in carbs you might be wondering where this fiber will come from.

First, grab a bunch of Asparagus from your local farmer's market. If they don't have any, then go to plan B, (the supermarket). Next, slice your Asparagus down the middle and toss it into a frying pan of bacon fat. While it's cooking add in a little salt, pepper or spice. There are no hard or fast rules with this, just keep trying new things until you find something you like. Once the Asparagus is softened put it on a plate and add a heaped tablespoon of sauerkraut. Bingo, your pro, and pre-biotics are ready to eat.

What did we learn from this?
The breakfast options in this section will outperform cereal or toast.

Homework: for some unique nutritional insight, check out this video by Dr. Berg. Paperback homies, you can find him on YouTube.
Link: https://www.youtube.com/watch?v=5vIoHR7J24I

Chapter 37

WHAT THE HELL DO I EAT FOR LUNCH?

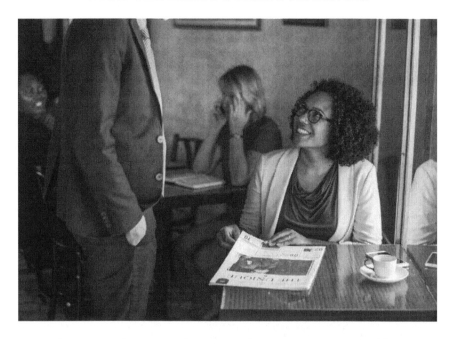

If you find yourself at work during lunchtime, your choices are eating out or taking a packed lunch. For those eating out, a word of caution – restaurants like to use bad fats because they are so cheap use.

So here's the golden rule. Whenever you find yourself eating out, take a second to look around at all the other folks frequenting your local food bar. If people look ill, then this isn't the watering hole for you. If there are lots of people jogging on the spot while wearing neon colored spandex, then you should be good to go.

Your other option is to take a packed lunch. It can actually be a great way to have more control over what you put into your belly. The key to making lunch work is to try to plan ahead. Remember the six P's. - Proper-planning-prevents-piss-poor-performance.

A packed lunch is best done the night before and then left in the fridge for morning. I know from personal experience, if it's not done the night before, it doesn't get done. Leaving everything until the last minute makes for a hungry, stressful day.

Again, I'm not trying to win any medals for cooking here, but I am aware that there is a whole generation who aren't used to preparing their own food. So the idea of this chapter is to get folks away from fast food. The ideas offered here are quick and inexpensive.

LAZY SALAD

Think of this first part as a "lazy salad" because it's so quick and easy to make. Simply grab a small Tupperware box and throw in a mixed salad. Let's not over think this one, you can add a few thinly sliced root vegetables like carrots, celery, onion etc. Bonus points if you can source these locally.

A handful of sprouted broccoli seeds is a good addition as are a few chopped olives. Before we close the lid sprinkle a little apple cider vinegar, Himalayan salt over the salad. A good way to increase the fat content is to add a little cold pressed olive oil. Just for good measure, you can also add a pinch of turmeric.

Tip – To make life easier, buy a $1 plastic spray bottle, remove the spray section and screw it directly onto the top of your vinegar bottle. It works like a charm and is perfect for evenly applying vinegar to salads.

So far we have invested maybe five minutes of the day preparing this. Keep coming, we are almost there. Now, let's add in a little protein.

If your budget is running tight you could easily add in any leftovers meat from the night before. Not too much mind, remember the ketogenic diet is about eating more meat, it's about trying to keep your ratio's balanced.

If you really are pressed for time, try sardines direct from the can. Unlike some other fish, sardines have enough selenium in them to counter any mercury found in the sea. If you do okay with them, you could easily switch things up with a boiled egg.

SOUP

If you really want to be ahead of the game bring a hot thermos flask. Homemade soup is super easy to make and it's something I'll cover in the next chapter. So far none of these ideas have included gluten.

DESERT

Fruit is good at kicking people out of ketosis. A workaround is to eat less of it. A Granny Smith apple has less sugar than most of those new hybrid apples. But it still has 14g of Carbohydrate. The solution? Cut it in half. Add a squirt of lemon juice to stop it from going brown (genetic modification not required).

You can boost the fat content by blending it up with cream of coconut – this comes in a can but be sure to get the one without any added sugar. If you feel the need to, add in a few berries from the lower end of the glycemic table, not too many mind.

Keep in mind that a banana has 27 g of total carbohydrate and 14 g of sugar. A better source of potassium is to pack an avocado instead. Avocado ticks the good fat, good fiber box and it's obviously lower in sugar.

If you find yourself getting hungry between meals, try nibbling on a small piece of ginger. Ginger will tame that snack attack. You can peel it on the fly quite easily by using the back of a spoon, no really, it's true.

KIDS LUNCH

Kids are funny – I should know, I used to be one. Ask any kid if they would like some sliced up coconut with cucumber and carrots dipped in hummus and they will inevitably say no. However, if you pay close attention you will notice that kids spend an inordinate amount of their time hanging off the fridge door complaining there is nothing to eat. Use this to your advantage.

Kids also like to see how far they can push you. If that's how your crew rolls, then you can even try a little reverse phycology. Here's how it works in three easy steps.

First: Know that kids are visual; if food is neatly cut up and arranged in bold colors they will be more tempted to try them. Second: placement is key, have the cut up vegetables placed at eye level in the fridge. Bonus points if you have brightly colored bowls to put them in. It may also help to have some form of healthy dip on hand too. Third: Tell your kids NOT to eat them. Sooner or later they will eat them – even if it's only to tell you how gross they are. I know right, getting a kid to eat healthily can be like negotiating with a terrorist.

Whatever you try, it helps to use a little imagination. But if this all seems like work, remember this is far easier than being held hostage to cook meals throughout the day. – And so far it's also been a pretty easy day for the dishwasher. Now you dunnit it.

Is it me, or is the dishwasher the only home appliance we make excuses for? Ask yourself, are really just "rinsing" those dirty dishes before putting them in the dishwasher? Or have we all been hoodwinked into doing the job we've paid the dishwasher to do? I digress.

NO GARDEN, NO PROBLEM

Imagine having a vegetable garden that produces clean nutrition year round. Imagine a garden with no weeding, no back-breaking digging, no bugs, no greenhouse, and not even any soil. And now imagine that the crops from this garden have a higher nutritional content than any whole food found in the supermarket! Better still, imagine that this crop can be grown within days on your kitchen counter. Best of all, it's incredibly cost-effective and simple to do.

Sprouts are something you can include in your lunchtime meals. It's actually so easy to do a child can do it – you catching my drift? Sprouting is a great way to get them to eat their healthy greens. This becomes easier and more fun when kids get to be part of the experiment.

Sprouted seeds are packed with nutrients and live enzymes. For sensitive individuals, sprouts can be a superior way to get your key nutrients rather than taking synthetic vitamins.

For the first couple of times, DON'T sprout more than a tablespoonful, this is a project you should grow into (yup, intended pun).

Here's a simple formula for sprouting:

• Buy (LARGE) seeds from a local store or a sprouting company online

• Soak the seeds

• Pour the seeds into a strainer

• Rinse every couple of hours

• Watch for tails to sprout from the seeds

• Keep rinsing to stop them from drying out

• Always check for mold

Sproutpeople.org is an online supplier that offers seeds along with more detailed information. The bulk of the information is given freely on their site.
If your system is fragile or just out of balance, sprouting can be a good way to get key nutrients into your body. Learning about sprouts can be a lot easier than learning about supplements.

Again, if this is all new to you, don't panic. A good rule of thumb is to simply fill 50% of every plate you serve yourself with green leafy vegetables. Do this one thing and you will be ahead of the pack.

What did we learn from this?
Thinking about meals ahead of time is the key to your success. Having something quick and easy that are prepared ahead of time can stop a snack attack in its tracks.

Homework: Check out montrealhealthygirl.com, or search for her videos on YouTube. Brittany has an extensive understanding of the healing process and she always manages to pack a few gems into her videos.

Chapter 38

WHAT THE HELL DO I EAT FOR DINNER?

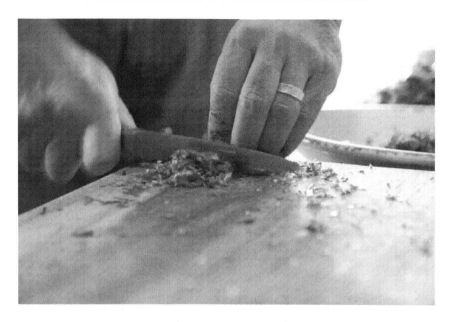

Straight out of the gate, any meal you attempt to cook is only as good as the ingredients you use. At this late point in the book, you should already have your local farmer on speed dial. Buying local is a great way to show your support for your local community.

If for some reason (?) you can't find a local farmer all is not lost. Today you can have grass-fed meat delivered directly to your door. How so?

For this tip, simply check out Butcher box.com; meat arrives fresh, sealed, and frozen via the miracle of dry ice. Once you have your basic materials the next step is to find the time to cook them. The good news is this chapter will show you how to cook your meals faster without the use of a microwave.

Look, we all know cooking a healthy meal from scratch is time-consuming. Enter the instant pot, a pressure cooker like no other! It takes all the pressure out of cooking. *No really, it's true.*

The instant pot can cook a meal 70% faster than regular cookers. If an instant pot before, then you are in for a pleasant surprise. It's a clever idea that gives you control over your kitchen. Hear me out on this one because even though pressure cookers have been around for a long time, this one recently went all electric. This not only made things easier, it also made pressure cooking safer. Hoorah for the instant pot.

As an added bonus pressure cookers reduce the lectin content of certain foods, this is something we covered earlier. For people like myself (without a lot of cooking skills) the Instant Pot is a game changer. You can literally throw food in an Instant Pot, walk away, and come back to a hot meal in half the time! Best of all you don't have to babysit the pot. It automatically turns off and then keeps the food warm until you are ready for it. In theory, you could throw the food in the morning, and it still is waiting for you ready to eat later that evening.

The Instant Pot is super simple to use hence it was the first kitchen appliance to ever go viral, and with zero advertising it quickly sold out.

If my wife ever decided to run off with my best friend (a) I'd sure miss him and (b) this is how I would feed myself until he came to his senses. lol.

There is an entire Instant Pot community on Facebook. I like to refer to them as potheads. Potheads offer lots of helpful recipes to get you started. The Instant Pot sells for around $99 on Amazon and comes with its own cookbook.

This offers good value for the money because it also doubles up as a slow cooker. What I like best about this idea is the instant pot has the added benefit of using a stainless steel pot. It's a win/win. As with any product I recommend, I've refrained from putting any direct links. That way, you can be sure I'm only recommending products that I believe will help you, as opposed to trying to profit from any kind of affiliated kick back. While we are on the subject, if you need a new blender, be sure to check out the "Blendtec", this bad boy is the absolute best!

HOMEMADE SOUP WITH A REGULAR SLOW COOKER

It took me a while to cross over to the instant pot. During that time, I was still cooking with a good old regular slow cooker. While obviously not as rock and roll as the instant pot, slow cookers are a useful tool to help get a hot meal on the table.

Here's a super easy way to make homemade chicken soup (trust me, even I struggle to get this one wrong). Preparing this meal takes maybe ten minutes. Doing it in the morning means you have a healthy hot meal to come home to. This style of cooking is real back-to-basics and pretty hard to mess up. As we move through the ingredients, you can obviously delete anything you are sensitive to.

For this example, simply place a whole chicken (preferably free range, local, or organic) into your instant pot (or slow cooker). Next, chop up and add a couple of onions and some vegetables. These can by anything you have on hand; maybe throw in some carrots, broccoli, celery, mushrooms, cabbage, garlic etc.

Add a teaspoon of Himalayan salt and even a few spices if you are feeling a tad rebellious. Almost done, now simply add enough water to cover the chicken and vegetable. If this is an instant pot just hit the button.

If it's a slow cooker turn it up high to get it cooking and then let simmer with the bones still in for a good few hours. If you have a low enough setting you can even let it simmer overnight, which adds to the flavor.

Once you are happy that the chicken has cooked, remove the bones and serve. That's it! The more times you make this meal the easier it gets. It's really not an exact science, just practice, eat and repeat.

Tip – You can also add a tablespoon of apple cider vinegar to the soup as it simmers. This will allow more minerals to leach out of the bones.

Obviously, cooking with pasture-raised, or wild caught meat generally increases the mineral count.

The chicken soup is a cost-effective meal that feeds a family of four twice over. Planning ahead is the key to a successful outcome. Waiting until you are hungry to figure out what's for dinner is a sure recipe for frustration.

BONE BROTH

Typically, bone broth is made using the bones of pasture-raised beef, lamb, pork, chicken, or even the heads of wild caught fish. Bone broth is best left simmering for a minimum of eight hours – but to get the most minerals out of bones, longer is better. Beef bones can cook for up to forty-eight hours. To help flood the broth with minerals, add vinegar to the water. While the bone broth simmers, you can also add your favorite herbs or vegetables to help make the taste more palatable. Once cooked, either sip on the liquid or use it as gravy poured over meals. You can even freeze any leftovers to give flavor to a later dish. Although you can certainly cook a bone broth on the stove top using a regular large pan, I find it easier to leave it in a slow cooker.

The amount of minerals found in bone broth is largely dependent on the quality of the bones. Finding bones from grass- or pasture-raised animals in your area is easy to do with a quick Google search.

Bone broth contains an abundance of the amino acids arginine, glycine, glutamine, and proline. These amino acids have powerful healing properties, especially for the lining of the gut. Bone broth is collagen-rich which may help to tighten the skin. Bone broth may also help alleviate joint pain.

If you don't have the time to make bone broth for yourself, Dr. Axe has an instant powdered bone broth that literally takes 5 minutes to make.

I hope something on these last three chapters has been useful to you. Obviously, these are just the basics that you can build up from. As you begin to grow in keto confidence be sure to check Leanne Vogel's book titled "The Keto Diet." It's beautifully designed, well written, and all her recipes are easy to follow.

What did we learn from this?
Cooking at home gives you greater control over what you eat. This is helpful for anyone with food sensitivities. Bone broths come loaded with minerals and amino acids which can help heal the gut.

Homework: to help keep this information balanced, watch this short video by Christa Orecchio. Christa's information is always clear, to the point and enjoyable to watch. Check out her link below.
https://thewholejourney.com/is-a-ketogenic-diet-good-or-bad

Chapter 39

REBUILD AND REPLENISH

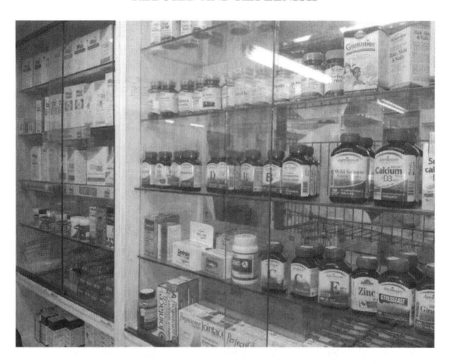

Our ancestors had the good sense to rotate crops which then gave the soil time to recover. Today we feed our crops fertilizers to make them grow faster. This results are more profitable crops for the large-scale farmer, but fewer minerals are found in the food.

Side by side, crops grown this way may look the same, but when the soil becomes mineral depleted the food becomes mineral deficient. Which in turn means that you become mineral deficient.
Think of it this way:

> Man owes his existence to a six-inch layer
> of topsoil and the fact that it rains. – Anonymous

Whatever minerals were found in farm soil fifty or even twenty-five years ago are no longer found in the soil today. As such, crops are more susceptible to bug infestations. Man's solution? Spray the crops with more poisons! *I know, right? You couldn't make this stuff up.*

Commercially grown crops have now become imposters of the real thing. They may look the same, but they are weaker than food once grown in nutrient dense soil. Perhaps we should think of soil as a bank account. If too much is taken out of it, the soil becomes bankrupt – and this is where we are today.

Our great grandparents had a simple solution. They knew that minerals could be added back into the soil by keeping old food scraps outside in a pile. Over time, these scraps would gradually decompose. This was then added back into the soil thus a cycle was created. A compost pile costs zero money to build and yet it's incredibly beneficial to the soil.

Supplementation can be a helpful tool for correcting any mineral imbalances in the body. Before we delve into this, let me first remind you that you cannot supplement your way out of a bad diet. And with a good diet, most people don't need supplements.
Given that we touched on this topic in an earlier chapter, I thought we could narrow this chapter down to five supplements worth trying.

MAGNESIUM

Magnesium makes it to the list because it covers so many bases. From head to toe magnesium is involved in more than 300 metabolic reactions! It can help with everything from normalizing blood pressure to keeping a steady heart rhythm. A lack of
magnesium can play a key role in anxiety and fatigue. It may surprise some to know that magnesium even plays a key role in the skeletal system!

A magnesium deficiency can occur for many reasons. It could be as a result of parasitic infection (hello again), a candida overgrowth (hello, hello), or as a result of a poor diet (hi). However, before you rush out to add it to your daily supplement routine it's worth knowing that there is more to magnesium supplementation than meets the eye.

For starters, there are nine common types of magnesium, all of which differ slightly in the benefits they offer. Also, magnesium *isn't* easily absorbed in pill form. If you are just starting out, try applying magnesium transdermally, which simply means applying it to the skin.

Another way to load up magnesium is by adding magnesium bath salts to your bath and soaking in them. Ideally, steer clear of products that add perfume to the ingredients.

VITAMIN B

B vitamins play an important role in keeping the body energized throughout the day. They also help to convert food into fuel.
B vitamin are sometimes offered as a complex. This usually includes B1, B2, B3, B5, B6, B7, B9 and sometimes B12.

B12 is a pretty big deal as it does so much in the body. Hence, it can also be purchased on its own. A B12 deficiency can leave a person feeling tired or unfocused. This may be coupled with a dizzy feeling or even heart palpitations. With so many overlapping symptoms, getting an accurate diagnosis can be particularly problematic.

Typically, a B12 deficiency is measured based on the serum vitamin B12 levels within the blood. But as we all know, standard blood tests allow some patients to fall through the cracks. A more precise screening might be one that checks for high homocysteine levels. Unfortunately, this test is usually only given to patients who have a known case of anemia or heart disease-related symptoms.

Sometimes doing things the old way by cross-checking a list of symptoms can prove just as helpful. Here's a list of things to be on the lookout for. An inability to concentrate, chronic fatigue, muscle weakness, joint pain, poor memory, heart palpitations, shortness of breath, dizziness, bleeding gums, a poor appetite and digestive problems.

A B12 deficiency may also have an impact on mood in the form of depression and anxiety.

The elderly become particularly prone to B12 deficiency. For anyone with relative showing signs of early dementia, adding a B-complex supplement may prove beneficial. A deficiency in B12 can also occur in someone who has absorption issues in the gut (hello again cheeky-leaky, fancy seeing you here).

Foods high in B12 are beef, chicken, liver, and fish such as wild caught salmon, herring, mackerel, and sardines. As such, many vegans may lean toward a B12 deficiency.

KRILL OIL

Krill oil is loaded with the omega-3 polyunsaturated fatty acids DHA (docosahexaenoic) and EPA (eicosapentaenoic acid). Both help keep the brain firing on all four cylinders. Krill oil is unique because unlike regular fish oils it can be absorbed directly by the brain with very little processing. It may also help support better concentration, memory, and learning.

Krill oil also has more antioxidants than regular fish oil and is generally considered safer because of its lower levels of contaminants such as mercury. Krill oil also contains astaxanthin which is helpful for the eyes. Given that the eyes have a high density of mitochondria; some reports suggest astaxanthin helps protect mitochondria from oxidative stress. *Hmm, I see.*

VITAMIN C

Vitamin C is a water-soluble vitamin, which simply means your body doesn't store it. Animals do have the ability to make vitamin C but oddly enough, we humans don't. Vitamin C made it to the list because it covers so many bases.

Vitamin C is a great go-to supplement whenever we feel a cold coming on. But the benefits of vitamin C can go well beyond supporting the immune system. It can be used to treat joint and muscle problems and it plays a role in a healthy heart. Yup, you heard me right on that last one. When it comes to the heart, vitamin C is right up there with healthy exercise.

Vitamin C is a powerful antioxidant, known to block some of the damage caused by DNA-damaging free radicals. Over time, free radical damage may accelerate aging and contribute to the development of heart disease. Vitamin C is useful in wound healing and skin health.

Vitamin C benefits the eyes and is thought to lower your risk of cataracts. Vitamin C supports the immune system and is important for respiratory health. Larger doses can be used for allergies and asthma due to its antioxidant and anti-inflammatory effect.

The brain and nervous system also have a need for vitamin C. Some sources suggest deficiencies can lead to a degeneration of the nervous system. Vitamin C even helps keep the tissue in the digestive tract healthy. It's useful for stomach ulcers, gastritis, and H. Pylori, (a bacterium known to cause chronic inflammation/infection in the stomach and duodenum).

The recommended daily allowance (RDA) for vitamin C has been established at 40 to 60 mg per day although some might suggest this is on the low end. Nobel Prize-winning scientist Linus Pauling, spent his life advocating amounts of 1,000 mg or even higher. He later died at the age of ninety-three. Higher doses of Vitamin C are sometimes administered by IV.

For anyone with an iron deficiency, pairing Vitamin C with iron has been shown to improve absorption. Pairing Vitamin C with the amino acid N-acetylcysteine (NAC) is an inexpensive way to help the body build glutathione, which I'm sure many of you already know is the body's master antioxidant.

PROBIOTICS:

Probiotics help increase the number of good bacteria found inside the gut. Some probiotics are best taken on an empty stomach and others require food, so be sure to read the label. As a rule of thumb, steer clear of bargain-priced probiotics.

Here are a few decent quality suppliers. Garden of life sells a good probiotic. As do Prescript-Assist which sells a probiotic that's made up of SBOs (soil based organisms). Standard Process has their pro-synbiotic. And Dr. Mercola sells a decent probiotic too.

These aren't the only options out there; I'm just trying to save you a little time. Ultimately it's important to find one that works for you. Some estimates suggest that 70% of the immune system lives in the gut. It should come as no surprise that probiotics improve immune function.

ADAPTOGENS

Adaptogenic herbs can help to bring a normalizing effect upon the body. Adaptogens are versatile and can be especially helpful when trying to balance out either Th1 or Th2 dominance.

Adaptogens can help increase the body's resistance to mental, physical, and environmental stress. That said, results will be hindered if the original stressor (i.e. food allergy) remains a constant. Earlier, we briefly mentioned Cordyceps which are not adaptogens (in the classic sense), but they do have adaptogenic qualities, hence they get a quick mentioned again here. Cordyceps can be helpful to those with adrenal stress.

What follows is a very basic summary of six widely used adaptogens. If this is all new to you, try to find an experienced herbalist to work with. *Okay, here we go.*

Ashwagandha has been used in Ayurvedic medicine for over 2000 years. Its immuno-modulating effects help the body adapt to stress. It can also be helpful in treating anxiety.

Ginseng is probably one of the more well-used adaptogens among herbalists. Asian ginseng is used most often because it is the most potent of the ginseng family. Studies show that Asian ginseng has great antioxidant effects, as well as helping your body adapt to stress. In some people, it can be helpful in lowering blood pressure.

Chaste Tree Berry (vitex agnus-castus) makes it to the list as it's especially helpful for the ladies. Chase tree mimics the master hormone, progesterone. Chaste tree can take up to eight weeks to feel the full effect, but once it kicks in, it can be a total game changer for many women.

Holy Basil helps fight fatigue and stabilize your immune system. It can also be used to regulate blood sugar and hormone levels.

Rhodiola is another potent adaptogen that helps the body adapt to stress-induced fatigue. Studies found that Rhodiola restores normal patterns of eating and sleeping brought on by long-term stress. It may also help to protect against oxidative stress, heat stress, radiation, and exposure to toxic chemicals. Some research suggests that Rhodiola can increases the use of oxygen and improve memory. It's also known to protect the heart and liver.

Gynostemma (or jiaogulan, as it's sometimes called) is a potent health tonic made as a tea. In addition to helping balance the immune system, Gynostemma also increases stamina as well as reducing stress. Gynostemma has a slightly woody taste which, given its health benefits, doesn't faze me in the slightest.

A WHOLE NEW YOU

Give the body the raw materials it needs and it will find a way to renew itself. It's sometimes said that every seven years we grow ourselves a whole new body! While there is some truth to this concept, our cells are constantly replacing themselves at varying rates. *Get this* ...

The lining of the stomach, for example, is replaced about every three days, while it's estimated that bones turn over every seven to ten years.

Our entire outer skin is replaced about every two weeks and the liver regrows itself every couple of years!

This cycle of events is not only remarkable it's actually a little freaky. Physically you are not the same person you were seven years ago. This presents a window of opportunity for anyone willing to make positive changes. **How well your body performs tomorrow is closely tied to the raw materials being used today.**

Even parts of your brain will regenerate, although not all. Some of us might warm to the idea of having a whole new brain; others will take comfort in knowing that essentially our memories remain the same.

As our time now draws closer to the end, I'm actually quite shocked at how much we managed to squeeze into one book. If there's anything I didn't cover, please feel free to let me know.

Finally, could you help me, please? As a new writer, I'm still trying to get my first 100 book reviews. If you enjoyed our time together, would you mind sharing your thoughts? *Thank you in advance.*

What did we learn from this?
Most people have some form of mineral deficiency. The right supplementation can help adjust the imbalance.

Homework: check out a website by the name of earthclinic.com. It is full of helpful tips, all presented in an easy to understand format. It also covers supplements and a wide range of ailments. I use this site often.

Link: https://www.earthclinic.com/

Chapter 40

RADICAL HOPE

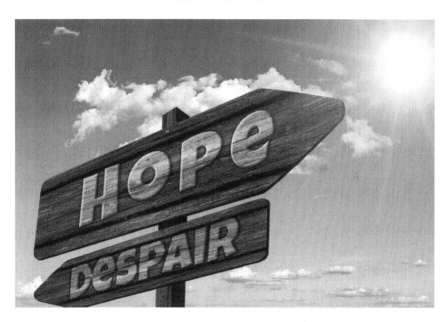

As we now begin our final descent I'm reflecting on the time we have spent together. For a book written primarily about health, we seem to have been on quite the journey.

At the beginning of this story, you found me trapped inside a wheelchair and unable to work. It's now been six years since I first became ill and seriously, as I type this draft, it's actually six years to the day!

While I'm thankful for all the things I have learned, it might surprise you to know that I'd trade them all in a heartbeat not to have gone through what I did. Forgive me if I appear ungrateful, but clawing back 95% of my health isn't something I choose to celebrate. Nope, today's ironic anniversary is all about the 5% that's stubborn remains, and how nobody has ever said "sorry."

Don't get me wrong, I'll take a 95% recovery over no recovery any day of the week. But to this day, I'm still forced to keep my symptoms in check. This takes effort on my part and I don't always have a lot of wiggle room.

My wife has often referred to me as the most persistent man she has ever met. I sometimes wonder what would have become of me had I *not* been so persistent? Perhaps at this moment, I'm seeing my glass as 5% empty, but I'm also thankful to be back on my feet and working again.

So far, I've narrowed the niggling problems that remain down to one of two things. Either my own understanding has reached its limitation, or the problem was intentionally made difficult to understand. What I do know for sure is this, after things went horribly wrong in 2011, I'm still the one picking up the pieces. God only knows what it was they introduced into my bloodstream but it *still* lurks deep inside me, albeit to a lesser degree.

Those times when I've used the term "God" in this book it's been my feeble attempt to describe whatever entity governs this vast universe. I find this concept more plausible than accepting we somehow grew legs and walked ourselves out of the sea.

That said, I don't think of myself as a religious person either. But the day I felt the coldness of death moving through my bones I happened to come across a small piece of scripture. I'd like to share it with you because something within this message gave me hope during a difficult time.

> *"For I know the plans I have for you," declares the Lord,*
> *"plans to prosper you and not to harm you,*
> *plans to give you hope and a future."*– Jeremiah 29:11

No matter *who* or *what* you believe in, there comes a point in this life when we are forced to accept our own mortality. When that day comes what we choose to think has the power to enslave or liberate us on the turn of a single thought. *How so?*

As someone who likes to be productive, the time I spent confined to a sickbed often left me feeling isolated. In some ways, being trapped by illness gave me a rare insight as to how an inmate might cope when forced to endure incarceration. At times the only places I got to visit were inside my head. Barren destinations that blew through my mind like a tumbleweed rolling across an open plain.

GATEWAY TO HEAVEN

However, one place I visited was quite different, and to this day it's held a lasting impression. In the middle of enduring much suffering, it was as if a gateway opened up deep in my subconscious.

I can still recall in quite vivid detail standing barefoot inside a small stone cottage located somewhere on a grassy hill. The smooth stone floor warmed with the amber glow of sunshine which filtered through a stained glass window. I've never lived in such a place but it immediately felt like home. Everything I touched had a distinctly natural feel to it, almost as if plastic and paint had never been invented.

Within that fleeting moment of peace and simplicity, it actually crossed my mind that perhaps my sickly body had given up and died. To be honest, wherever it was that I'd found myself, I was in no rush to leave.

Snapping back to reality left me reluctantly pondering the meaning of such a detailed image. Maybe I'd caught a glimpse of how we were supposed to live – in the moment, simply, and free of worry rather than chasing every dollar. I guess some parts of this book were inspired by that blissful feeling. Others were written to address the inadequacies of a medical establishment that left me out to dry.

THE WHEEL OF MISFORTUNE

Over the years I've had my share of troubles and I suspect you have had yours too. That ugly wheel of misfortune can be such an unpredictable part of life. We all have "character building" days – you know the ones I'm talking about, those days when you lose your job and your car keys in the same afternoon. Unfortunately, bad days aren't limited to losing replaceable things, although that sucks too.

Bad things happen to good people all of the time and none of us are immune. Maybe you already know what it's like to lose someone close to you, or perhaps you know what it's like to suffer from medical injury or be a victim of a crime. While our past certainly shapes us, it doesn't have to define who we are. For just a moment, I'd like to ask you to pause here, set down the book, and let your mind briefly drift back to one of your more challenging days.

WHAT WOULD YOU SAY?

I can only imagine where your mind went to and how that unfortunate day might have impacted your life. I wonder, if you again had the opportunity to travel backward in time and were somehow able to stand next to yourself, what words of wisdom would you whisper in your ear?

If I could go back in time, I'd tell myself, be still and know that in the end, it's going to be okay, just don't lose hope. When a storm rain's down on us, we don't always need to know the reason why; we just need to know it's going to be okay. It's as if our earthly soul needs something tangible to hold onto, perhaps just a small flicker of hope to reignite our human spirit. When we are deprived of such hope the world becomes a daunting place.

> To be truly radical is to make hope possible
> rather than despair convincing. – Raymond Williams

You may have noticed how in recent times the word "hope" became part of a political slogan. The word was hyped up and bandied around with broad smiles and a promise that we all wanted to believe in. You may have also noticed that political hope rarely reaches the bottomless pit of human despair. Stay with me here, because even though those damned spin doctors hijacked the word hope, it's vitally important they aren't allowed to keep it. *Come, let's travel down one last road together...*

Over the years, I've come to understand that the vast majority of people on this planet all want the same things that you and I do, meaningful work, someone who believes in them, and hope. Nobody wakes up and asks, "How can I make my life hopeless today?" Nope, that circumstance is usually imposed on us by men in suits – but it doesn't have to be this way.

Look beyond those daily news headlines and you will notice that most of us are simply just trying to get by. Not everyone is an ax-wielding maniac, although there are some that are. Not everyone is out to deceive you, although there are some that will. But if we put our humanitarian goggles on for just a second perhaps we can see that people are a product of their environment. It's been my observation that **those who make the worst choices are the ones with the least amount of options.** It's much easier to be an upstanding citizen with a $100 bill in your pocket than it is with an empty purse and kids to feed. *I digress.*

You and I were not made to be dumb creatures. In case it escaped your attention, we are the only mammals on this planet currently driving around in cars. And yet when the human brain is flooded with stress and toxins we all have a tendency to make dumb mistakes. *Okay, where am I heading with this?*

Having seen a very different world, albeit briefly, I believe that simplicity and gratitude are significantly undervalued. Alas, the darkness created in this world keeps us rooted in greed and indifference. But it's this same darkness that helps us see the brightness of the light. *Check this out ...*

As rational thinkers, it can be difficult to understand how we can benefit ourselves by helping others. But I wouldn't be wasting your time or mine if I hadn't experienced the value of this firsthand. What I'm about to tell you will have a huge health benefit. *Ready?*

HACK YOUR ATTITUDE WITH GRATITUDE

Gratitude has a profound effect on the mind, body, and soul. Gratitude has been shown to turn off stress, blast away critical thinking and wipe away selfishness. Gratitude can even turn off that most destructive of all human conditions – a victim mentality.

If you want to take your health to a whole different level, learn to give freely and be grateful for the experience. *But what does that even mean, and how do we do it?*

First, you can just go ahead and relax, if counting your money with fingerless gloves on is your thang, that's okay. This final health tip will work with or without money.

Giving something back is a powerful tool to have under your health belt, *no really, it's true.* It can be as profound as saving a life or as simple as helping someone across the road. At this point, it's important *not* to let the simplicity of this concept undermine your perception.

EXPECT NOTHING

Let's take a step back and look at this from a fresh angle. You can take it to the bank that right now there is someone out there who is experiencing a soul-crushing day, the depths of which you and I can only imagine. How would you like to become an intrinsic part of *their* story and in the process *you* get to reap the health rewards? The trick to doing this is to expect nothing in return. Once you get to that level, something freaky happens. Giving freely opens the path to receiving. Stay with me here, I promise this final tip has a great deal of science behind it.

Back when I was too ill to work there were people in my local community who did something that to this day still blows me away. Without being asked they pitched in and started to leave prepaid gas cards and grocery cards in my mailbox. This act of generosity came with no strings attached at a time when I felt had no value.

I later learned that some of those people who gave had never met me in person and yet they still chose to help. Although the money quickly came and went, those envelopes represented *more* to me than just food and gasoline. In my darkest hour, it was as if someone gently whispered in my ear, *it's going to be okay – so don't give up.*

374

Six years later those random acts of kindness remain firmly rooted inside me. That selfless, bright light of humanity continues to chase away the darkness of greed. *So where does all this fit in?*

Let's go back to that bad day *you* were having, maybe you did lose your car keys and your job in the same afternoon. On that lousy bus ride home how would you feel if suddenly you found an envelope on your seat? Inside that envelope, there was no note, just a few dollars, perhaps only enough to buy yourself dinner at the end of a long miserable day. I know, right? WTF? (Who's-This-From?)

Suddenly in the middle of a storm of shit, this becomes an almost surreal single ray of sunshine. In the absence of any note, you'd be forced to ponder the meaning of it all. But *how* the heck would that envelope find you on that bus, and *why?*

Here's the how.

Stop for just a second and look up from your phone. People are hurting all around, they really aren't that difficult to find. Right now there is someone close to you that's struggling to keep their heads above water as I once was.

To see someone who's genuinely in need and then, *without* drawing attention to yourself, be prepared to step in and help is a beautiful thing. But this is far more than just a gesture of goodwill, it's a symbol of **hope.** *But how can this increase your health?*

GETTING HIGH

There's actually a whole mountain of published scientific data that points to how we can lift ourselves by lifting others. No, seriously, this is sometimes referred to as "Helper's-High." Don't take my word for it, once you finish this final chapter you can easily find a mountain of data on sites such as PubMed.

One study showed that helping others led to a measurable increase in longevity. Just think back to that remarkable 102-year old lady Eddie Simms, she spends her days helping "younger" members of the nursing home.

Another study showed a measurable decrease in pain! But here's the biggy. One study showed that people who observe feats of generosity are more likely to do the same. Thus causing a ripple effect throughout an entire community. *Wait a second, are you getting this?*

When one person performs a good deed, it literally causes a chain reaction of other altruistic acts! Think about it, this world has become a breeding ground for habitual greed, and materialism. And yet these are the very things that steal our inner peace.

If the secret to living is giving, then your mission from today on is a simple one: be a tiny symbol of hope to someone and in the process boost your own health!

PERSISTENCE

Over the course of this book, we have crammed quite a few tools into our proverbial toolbox. But our old friend persistence remains my favorite, if for no other reason than it displays total disobedience in the face of adversity.

Persistence is nothing more than exhausting all other options and then finding a way to try just one more. Persistence is believing that all problems have solutions, just as doors have keys. Persistence is simply a case of finding ways to move sideways when the road ahead becomes blocked. Persistence helped me write this book.

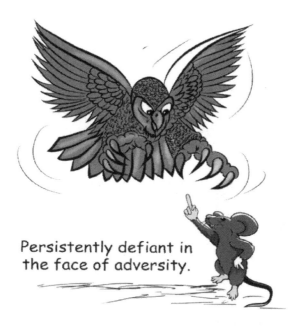

Persistently defiant in
the face of adversity.

Throughout our time together, I've always tried to keep things real.
I've never pretended to be something that I'm not, or to have all
the answers. *I'm not sure anybody does.* At best, discovery is a
collective effort and a great starting point is to always be reading
something new.

I first began applying the techniques in this book back in 2013/14
and I have more I'd like to share with you. But for the moment, my
time isn't always my own.

As I write this, I'm currently working for a small masonry firm out
of Boston. And while construction work pays my rent, it sadly cuts
into my writing time. Do I want to be pushing a wheelbarrow
around when I'm pushing sixty? *Nope, I do not.*

Some days I feel the need to write like some people need air. So much so, that I've been spending my weekends writing a small handbook titled "Heavy Metals Detox."

I felt this was an important topic in desperate need of simplification. At times, many of the experts who understand the scope of this problem might as well talk in a foreign language. I've managed to buffer all that complex information and **present it in a way that is not only helpful, but it's also enjoyable to read.**

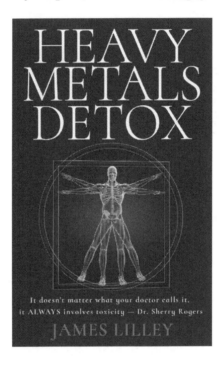

The challenge for me *isn't* finding things to write about, it's trying to get noticed in a sea of other books. I'm currently thinking of putting an ad in the local paper that reads, "Handyman – will write for food" lol.

I guess my career as a writer depends on how well *this* book is received. I accept that my style is a little different from the norm. While some might find it oddly refreshing, others might not be able to see past my new author label. Who knows, perhaps next time I'll try my luck writing in a different genre.

Either way, it's been my absolute pleasure writing for you. When I started on this path it was always my intention to create at least one book worthy of reading. I hope I have achieved that standard for you.

Before I crawl back under my rock, may I ask for a small favor of you? With no slick, million-dollar marketing team behind me, good old fashioned word of mouth is my preferred way to advertise. If you enjoyed this book, would you please leave a review or give it a shout somewhere on social media? Platforms such as Goodreads, Pinterest, Facebook, or Instagram are perfect.

As our story now draws to a close, I'm also aware of how fickle the outside world can be. I find the words of Elbert Hubbard offer some comfort: **"To avoid criticism, do nothing, say nothing, and be nothing."**

For what it's worth, I actually gave this book my all, and anything less would have been a wasted effort. So for now, I guess that's it, except to say thank you for your valued support and good luck on your own journey.

Author gently sets down the pen and quietly leaves the room. *I know, right? Dropping the mic would have been a tad pretentious.*

Kindest Regards
James.

Oh yeah, one last thing,
Dad, if you can somehow see me,
I miss your face

and I dedicate this book to you.

Your support for an indie author is greatly appreciated.

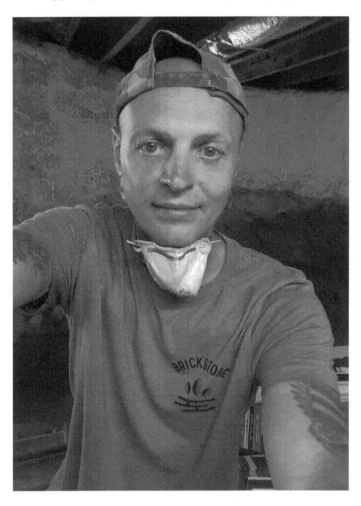

It should come as no surprise that I don't have any slick photos of myself in the bathroom mirror while wearing green spandex. *I'm still a working man trying to get through the day, but at night, writing brings me alive!*

SPECIAL THANKS TO

To Amanda, who always believed in my ability to write this book. I know this past year hasn't always been easy, but here we both are at the finish line. Thank you for your unwavering support.

Miss Emma, thank you for your contributions, your letter was quite moving. I suspect you will one day be great writer that people will flock to read. To the one and only Miss Abigail, your presence always makes me smile. Jade- thank you for always bigging me up. For sure, Grandad would be so proud of you.

To my old friend Steve Shaw, whom I've always trusted to always tell me like it is. To Dalton Lawrence, your true value in this life that has yet to be realized.

Finally, to all the many health gurus featured in this book, I've learned so much from each and every one of you. I'm truly grateful for the good work that you do.

Thank you.

2017
My beautiful wife Amanda, who I managed to send grey.

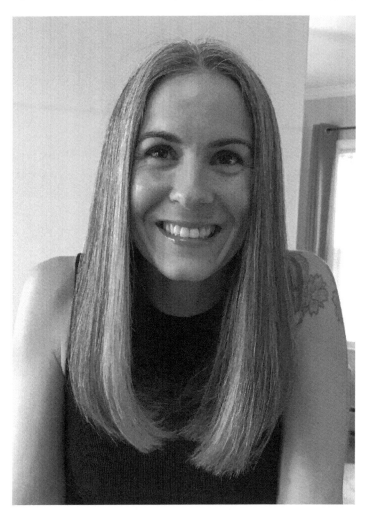

You can check out Amanda's stunning
knitting patterns on Ravelry.com

Your voice is powerful

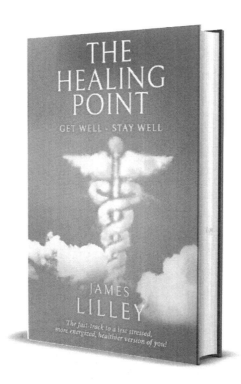

Please share it!

S.O.S

I could use a little help

Here's the problem. For whatever reason, some of my reviews aren't getting through (see below).

 Lori Pena For some reason my Kindle wouldn't let me give a Amazon review!! It is an amazing book!! I love the stories about your Dad. Reading it over again today. Thank you!!!

Sad · Reply · 2w 3

 Michelle Callaghan I also cannot leave any reviews..

Sad · Reply · 2w 1

Beverley McCullagh Same here

Like · Reply · 5d

To be honest, I find this a little discouraging. Reviews offer social proof that this book has a value. On the flip side, whenever someone shares my book on social media it brings a huge smile to my face. *No really, it's true!*

Your voice powerful, please use it. Many thanks.

Back in 2014 very few people had heard of the word "Ketogenic". I was considered a bit of an oddball doing some "crazy keto thing." Today low carb, high fat diets have become mainstream. I've always enjoyed being ahead of the curve, learning new things and putting theories to the test.

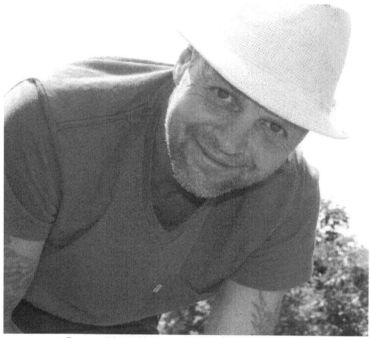

James 2014 (doing some crazy keto thing)

I'm currently trying something new. The past few months, I've been intentionally keeping myself out of ketosis. Some of the things I'm doing may surprise you, and I'm pretty sure some of it would shock you to the core!

MORE STUFF KALE SOUP CAN'T FIX

During my time in construction I see plenty of toxic homes that no amount of kale soup is going to fix. Damp and mold are good examples of this. All too often, homeowners are given the *wrong* advice or sold products they simply don't need.

But with the *right* approach damp and mold are relatively easy to fix. If enough folks are looking for answers, perhaps I'll write a short handbook for making homes less attractive to mold.

If you need help in this area you can always shoot me a message via my FB page, here's the link

https://www.facebook.com/james.lilley.393950
.

James - Dislikes selfies, (likes reviews)

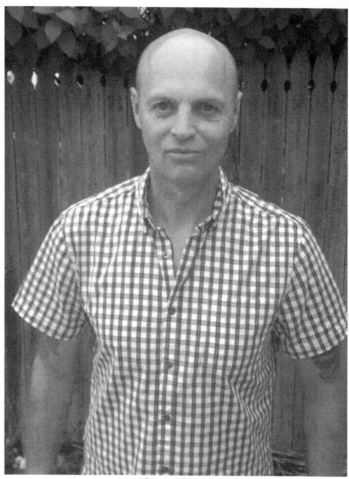

James 2017

It makes me happy that you read this book. But as someone who *dislikes* attention, I would rather **not** have my photo taken. I'm here taking a hit for the team as a way of saying thanks to those folks who took time out of their busy day to leave a review.

SET IT FREE!

If this is a paperback copy, it's been read, you don't need it, *and someone else just might.*

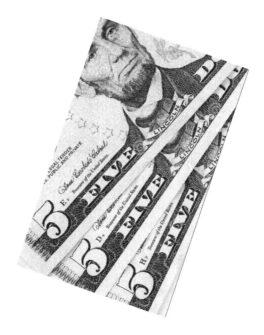

Consider leaving a copy in the most random place you can think of perhaps with a five-dollar bill inside left as a bookmark. **Let the finder experience a totally random act of kindness,** and maybe in turn they will do the same!

Depression, fatigue, insomnia, anxiety, brain fog, weakness, **it doesn't matter what your doctor calls it, it ALWAYS involves toxicity** — Dr. Sherry Rogers.

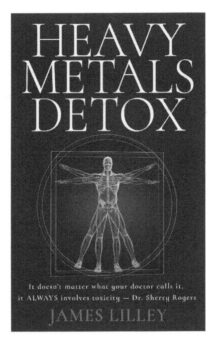

Rest assured, this book contains everything you need to keep your health on track. Inside, we'll cover what heavy metals are, how they get inside us, and what you can do to remove them.

When **aluminum, mercury, lead, arsenic, cadmium, and chromium** are gently purged from the body, a stronger, clearer-thinking version of YOU comes to the surface. As an added bonus, detoxification helps protect against accelerated aging and sickness.

In 1974 the World Health Organization reported that **82%** of all chronic degenerative disease was caused by toxic metal poisoning! Since then, heavy metals have continued to find their way into our food, our water, and even the air we breathe!

When doctors fail him, James turns to natural medicine and whole foods. Today he is well. From wheelchair to wellness this remarkable story is the blueprint he used to spearhead his recovery.

Here's a snapshot of what's inside...

- How to quickly find the root cause of symptoms
- Overcome chronic pain without popping pills
- The importance of sleep and how to do it right
- How to rid the body of heavy metals, parasites, and fungi
- Know which supplements promote health (and which to avoid)
- Where to find the cleanest foods (spoiler alert, they *aren't* in the organic section)
- How to curb unhealthy food cravings
- Effective techniques that tackle stress, insomnia, and fatigue
- Know what to eat and when to eat it *without* feeling overwhelmed or confused
- Proven techniques that boost energy
- Finally, say goodbye to brain fog and hello to mental clarity

The fast-track to a less stressed, more energized, healthier version of YOU!

For people who read from the back,
hello to you - here's what you missed

> # You don't need to spend thousands of dollars to be healthy, you just need to be able to read.
>
> James Lilley

Thank you and goodnight
James

NOTES

NOTES

Made in the USA
San Bernardino, CA
05 August 2019